THE EXPERIENCE OF HEARING LOSS

Hearing loss is a common chronic condition which is often poorly recognized but can have multiple negative impacts, not just on the lives of those directly affected, but also those living with them. People with impaired hearing may begin a long and uncertain journey involving a number of key stages, from emerging awareness and help-seeking, to diagnosis, adjustment, and self-evaluation.

Based on a model of person-centered audiological rehabilitation, this book explains why it is important to understand both patients' own experiences, and those of their communication partners, over time. It focuses particularly on the human dynamics of hearing loss, exploring the broader consequences of hearing loss for the individual, family members, and wider society. In particular the book:

- gives insight into the patients' and their communication partners' experiences and perspectives through clear and telling first-hand narrative accounts;
- examines how people understand their own hearing loss, reflect on their experiences with hearing aids – both positive and negative – and evaluate treatment options;
- considers the changes needed to conversations in order to include all communication partners, whether with impaired hearing or not; and
- discusses consequences of hearing loss using the International Classification of Functioning, Disability and Health (ICF).

With its explicit aim to increase awareness of the need to include the patient and close relatives in the process of rehabilitation, this new text makes an important contribution to further improve evidence-based practice in the field of audiological rehabilitation. An ideal text for audiology, ENT, and nursing students of all levels.

Vinaya Manchaiah is Jo Mayo Endowed Professor in the Department of Speech and Hearing Sciences at Lamar University, USA. He is also the co-founder of the not-for-profit and non-governmental organization Audiology India.

Berth Danermark is Professor of Sociology in the School of Health and Medical Sciences at Örebro University, Sweden. He is the director of doctoral studies at the Swedish Institute for Disability Research.

THE EXPERIENCE OF HEARING LOSS

Journey through aural rehabilitation

Edited by Vinaya Manchaiah and
Berth Danermark

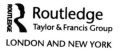

Routledge
Taylor & Francis Group

LONDON AND NEW YORK

First published 2017
by Routledge
2 Park Square, Milton Park, Abingdon, Oxon OX14 4RN

and by Routledge
711 Third Avenue, New York, NY 10017

Routledge is an imprint of the Taylor & Francis Group, an informa business

British Library Cataloguing in Publication Data
A catalogue record for this book is available from the British Library

Library of Congress Cataloguing in Publication Data
Names: Manchaiah, Vinaya, editor. | Danermark, Berth, 1951– editor.
Title: The experience of hearing loss: journey through aural rehabilitation /
[edited by] Vinaya Manchaiah and Berth Danermark.
Description: Milton Park, Abingdon, Oxon; New York, NY: Routledge, 2017. |
Includes bibliographical references.
Identifiers: LCCN 2016031281| ISBN 9781138642201 (hardback) |
ISBN 9781138642225 (pbk.) | ISBN 9781315630090 (ebook)
Subjects: | MESH: Hearing Loss – rehabilitation | Quality of Life |
Correction of Hearing Impairment | Adult
Classification: LCC RF291 | NLM WV 270 | DDC 617.8–dc23
LC record available at https://lccn.loc.gov/2016031281

ISBN: 978-1-138-64220-1 (hbk)
ISBN: 978-1-138-64222-5 (pbk)
ISBN: 978-1-315-63009-0 (ebk)

Typeset in Bembo
by Out of House Publishing

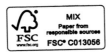

Printed and bound in Great Britain by
TJ International Ltd, Padstow, Cornwall

CONTENTS

FIGURES

TABLES

CONTRIBUTORS

Ann-Christine Gullacksen, Ph.D.

Former Associate Professor of the Faculty of Health and Society, Malmö University, Sweden. Within a social science approach, Dr. Gullacksen's main focus in research has been issues related to patient and user perspectives on rehabilitation. She has primarily studied psychosocial consequences for persons living with hearing disabilities and persons affected by chronic pain. She has also been involved in developing a model for participatory dialogue to be used in meetings between patients, users, and professionals.

Berth Danermark, Ph.D.

Professor of Sociology at Örebro University, Sweden. Co-founder of and Director of doctoral studies at the Swedish Institute for Disability Research. Within the field of disability research, Prof. Danermark focuses primarily on issues related to hearing and communication from a social, psychological, and psychosocial perspective. In collaboration with researchers in other disciplines, he has developed an interdisciplinary approach that interweaves a behavioral and social science perspective both technically and medically. Prof. Danermark is also currently working on issues related to inter-professional collaboration.

Calum Delaney, Ed.D.

Senior Lecturer and Head of Speech and Language Therapy, Centre for Speech and Language Therapy & Hearing Science, Cardiff Metropolitan University, Wales, United Kingdom. In relation to audiology and speech-language pathology practice, Dr. Delaney has an interest in clinical decision-making, and the communication that takes place between client and clinician in the clinical context.

Fei Zhao, M.D., Ph.D.
Principal Lecturer in Audiology, Centre for Speech and Language Therapy & Hearing Science, Cardiff Metropolitan University, Wales, United Kingdom. Guest Professor at the School of Hearing and Speech Sciences, Sun Yat-sen University in China. Dr. Zhao's research theme is dedicated to providing better hearing health care and prevention, together with improving the inclusion of people with hearing impairment.

Hans Henrik Philipsen, Ph.D.
Chief consultant on Innovation & Development for the Ida Institute, Denmark. He applies his expertise as a Social Anthropologist to better understand the challenges and opportunities facing modern hearing care. His ethnographic videos are widely used in the education of hearing care professionals worldwide.

Joseph Montano, Ed.D.
Associate Professor of Audiology and Director of Hearing and Speech at Weill Cornell Medical College in New York City, USA. His clinical interests include adult audiologic rehabilitation, counseling, and amplification. He is currently the ASHA Vice President for Standards and Ethics in Audiology and Past President of the Academy of Rehabilitative Audiology. He serves on the advisory boards for Hearing Education and Awareness for Rockers (HEAR) and the Hearing Rehabilitation Foundation. In addition to numerous presentations and publications, he is the co-editor of the book *Adult Audiologic Rehabilitation.*

Lindsey E. Jorgensen, Au.D., Ph.D.
Assistant Professor, Department of Communication Sciences and Disorders, University of South Vermillion, South Dakota, USA. Within the field of auditory rehabilitation research, Dr. Jorgensen focuses primarily on issues related to hearing and communication, and the use of hearing assistive technology in normal aging and cognitive impairment. She teaches Doctor of Audiology students both in didactic coursework and clinically. Additionally, she conducts research and clinical work for the Department of Veterans Affairs.

Margaret Nowak, B.S.
Current Doctor of Audiology student at Rush University, Chicago, Illinois, USA. Ms. Nowak is primarily interested in the areas of adult audiological rehabilitation and electrophysiology. She has presented locally and nationally on the complex rehabilitative interventions of aging individuals with dual sensory impairment.

Marieke Pronk, Ph.D.
Hearing health scientist and epidemiologist, postdoctoral researcher at the Department of Otolaryngology – Head and Neck Surgery, Ear & Hearing, VU University Medical Center and the EMGO⁺ Institute, Amsterdam, the Netherlands. Dr. Pronk is also a team member of the Longitudinal Aging Study Amsterdam. Her research is characterized by an epidemiological and longitudinal approach and focuses on the broad field of hearing loss in aging older adults. Her current main fields of interest are: psychosocial

consequences of hearing loss, factors influencing hearing help-seeking and hearing aid uptake, and longitudinal change in hearing loss.

Mariska Stam, Ph.D.

Hearing health scientist and epidemiologist, postdoctoral researcher at the Department of Otolaryngology – Head and Neck Surgery, Ear & Hearing, VU University Medical Center and the EMGO⁺ Institute, Amsterdam, the Netherlands. Dr. Stam's research incorporates the broad field of hearing epidemiology. In particular, she is interested in the prospective impact of hearing impairment on various aspects of life (e.g., participation in work, psychosocial health, comorbidity) of adults.

Melanie Gregory, M.Sc.

Senior audiologist at the Ida Institute, which aims to foster better understanding of human dynamics of hearing loss. The focus of her work is promoting a person-centered approach in hearing care through developing think-tank innovation processes and counselling resources. She considers that the patent's perspective or journey is the starting point for process and resource development. She has contributed significantly to implement the patient–centered care within audiology by training audiologists across the globe.

Patricia McCarthy, Ph.D.

Professor in Audiology, Associate Chair and Au.D. Program Director, Department of Communication Disorders and Sciences, Rush University, Chicago, Illinois, USA. Prof. McCarthy's research, writing, national and international presentations, and teaching have focused on adult audiological rehabilitation.

Rebecca Kelly-Campbell, Ph.D.

Audiology Postgraduate Coordinator, Department of Communication Disorders, University of Canterbury, Christchurch, New Zealand. Dr. Kelly-Campbell's teaching and research interest are in adult audiologic rehabilitation, with a focus on non-hearing aid management strategies for adults with hearing problems.

Samuel Trychin, Ph.D.

Licensed psychologist specializing in the cognitive, emotional, physical, and social effects of less than normal hearing. Dr. Trychin has developed and adopted a variety of effective tactics and strategies to prevent or reduce its negative effects. He has presented this information internationally. He is a currently a member of the Governor's Advisory Council for Deaf and Hard of Hearing and a member of the Governor's Advisory Council on Aging in the Commonwealth of Pennsylvania. He is also Academy Curriculum Consultant to the Hearing Loss Association of America (HLAA).

Sapna Mehta, Au.D.

Clinical audiologist at Weill Cornell Medicine in New York, USA, where Dr. Mehta is clinically involved in the diagnosis of hearing and balance disorders, and in the management of hearing loss and tinnitus. Her interests lie in the assessment of aural rehabilitation interventions, including hearing aids, cochlear implants, and auditory training.

Sarah Granberg, Ph.D.
The Swedish Institute for Disability Research (SIDR), School of Health Sciences, Örebro University, Sweden and Audiological Research Centre, Örebro University Hospital, Sweden. Dr. Granberg works as a lecturer in Audiology and as a researcher in disability research with a special interest in hearing loss. Her current research concerns adults with hearing loss and the International Classification of Functioning, Disability, and Health (ICF), and older adults with Dual-Sensory-Loss (DSL).

Sophia E. Kramer, Ph.D.
Professor in Auditory Functioning and Participation at the VU University Medical Center in Amsterdam, the Netherlands. Prof. Kramer holds a University Research Chair and is a co-director of the Quality of Care program of the EMGO Institute for Health and Care Research. She is mainly involved in research activities, but also engaged in clinical work. Her research focuses on the psychosocial and cognitive effects of adult hearing impairment and the development of methods to assess these effects. This includes the assessment of listening effort using pupillometry. Prof. Kramer served as president of the International Collegium of Rehabilitative Audiology (2011–2013). In 2016, she received the International Award in Hearing from the American Academy of Audiology.

Vinay Swarnalatha Nagaraj, Ph.D.
Professor of Audiology, Norwegian University of Science and Technology, Norway. Prof. Nagaraj has academic qualifications from All India Institute of Speech and Hearing, India and Cambridge University, UK. He is a member of the working group in the European Federation of Audiological Societies for school-age hearing screening.

Vinaya Manchaiah, Au.D., MBA, Ph.D.
Based in the Department of Speech and Hearing Sciences, Lamar University, Beaumont, Texas, USA and holds the following positions: Director of Audiology, Jo Mayo Endowed Professor, and Associate Professor of Audiology. Dr. Manchaiah has worked in various clinical, teaching, research, and administrative roles. He has served as the Board of Director of the British Academy of Audiology and the President of an NGO – Audiology India, which he co-founded. His main research interest is in adult audiological rehabilitation.

Wenlong Xiong, M.D.
Centre for Speech and Language Therapy & Hearing Science, Cardiff Metropolitan University, Wales, United Kingdom. Dr. Xiong graduated from China Medical University, and earned his Master's degree at the Peking Union Medical University, China. He is currently studying the topic of "Patient-Centred Care in Audiological Rehabilitation."

FOREWORD

The need for adult aural rehabilitation (AR) was recognized in the United States some 70 years ago, and originated because of the large number of soldiers with hearing loss returning home. At that time, veterans with service-related hearing loss benefitted from a residential program at one of three strategically located hospitals across the USA, where a comprehensive six-week program provided by a multidisciplinary team was carried out involving audiologists, speech pathologists, psychologists, and otologists. The services they received emphasized speech and lip-reading, listening exercises (auditory training), and the fitting of hearing aids (extremely primitive in comparison to today). In no other time or place since then has AR received so much focus and attention; this was the worldwide "heyday" for AR. It is important to realize, however, that the veterans who participated in this innovative effort had no choice – after all, they were soldiers following orders.

Unfortunately, we who have experienced much of the journey that audiology has traveled since then have seen how AR services have not been embraced. Despite multiple textbooks on the subject and "lip service" about how AR is needed for successfully overcoming the challenges of auditory disability, few audiology practitioners provide structured AR programs to their patients on a regular basis. In fact, in the USA, reimbursement is not available to compensate for the time that audiologists spend providing AR services.

However, the winds are shifting. Audiology research and rehabilitation is again focusing on the importance and value of AR. Increasingly, we are being reinforced by research findings and clinical experiences that show the significant benefits and improvements derived from structured AR being provided to our patients. The basic premise is the same as it was long ago – to achieve the best possible outcome through a comprehensive program tailored for each patient. However, the principles and guidelines are vastly different, because it is now known that AR encompasses the development of a wider set of activities and skills, and the focus is to improve all abilities that contribute to understanding spoken language. With this new definition and conceptual framework, there are new approaches involving: visual aspects of communication, controlling background noise, attending to linguistic cues, developing repair strategies, applying assertive techniques, improving and situating proper positioning and lighting, eliciting the cooperation of communication partners, and a host of others. All of these aspects are covered in this text.

As the new awareness for AR is becoming more recognized, the number of publications in scholarly journals is increasing exponentially, and there have been several excellent recent AR textbooks for adults and children. Most of the work and publications has taken a clinician/research viewpoint; such work has had an "extrinsic" rather than "intrinsic" or "introspective" focus. That is, for years AR programs have taken a clinical/research view – how to approach the process as a practitioner or researcher. This perspective is important, but is severely limited because it fails to recognize the value and importance of the most critical components of the process: patients and their significant others. This unique aspect is what makes this text by Drs. Manchaiah and Danermark so different. These authors and editors have deftly focused on the introspective perspective of AR with a patient/communication partner approach. This is analogous to the now well-recognized, well-tested process of including the consumer in developing advertising campaigns to attract and entice them to purchase a product. It is clear that this process really, really works, otherwise product advertising would not be a multimillion dollar industry.

Another unique aspect of this text is reflected in the title that includes the word "journey." A journey is a trip, it is a passage or travel from one place or stage to another, and reflects exactly what the AR process involves in order to be successful. The journey begins with initial identification or recognition of auditory disability, and the endpoint is the time of acceptance of how to live with and maximize communication in view of the inability to hear or process sound. In addition to Drs. Manchaiah and Danermark, excellent authors were chosen for each chapter based on their publication and clinical experience of the variety of topics covered by the text.

Those interested in AR and how to entice those who would benefit from a structured AR program will be more than pleased with this text. It provides the basis for delivering AR programs to those in need of therapy in a highly effective, unique way that allows the clinicians to bring AR into the limelight it so aptly deserves.

Ross J. Roeser, Ph.D.
Lois and Howard Wolf Professor in Pediatric Hearing
Executive Director Emeritus
University of Texas at Dallas
Callier Center for Communication Disorders
Dallas, Texas, USA

PREFACE

For large numbers of people, hearing loss occurs gradually. In the beginning, problems related to the hearing difficulty may only be occasional, but eventually increase to a stage where it significantly interferes with life. Consequences of hearing loss may extend to family members, friends, and colleagues. Moreover, hearing-loss related experiences of all those affected may change over time. It is noteworthy that very little attention has been paid to how these experiences change with time and what factors and mechanisms trigger these changes. Better understanding of such aspects will provide unique insight into the human dynamics associated with hearing loss.

The Ida Institute, based in Denmark, initially proposed the idea of a *patient journey*. The institute is an independent, non-profit organization with the vision to foster a better understanding of the human dynamics of hearing loss. They believe in interdisciplinary collaborative work to develop various tools that foster patient-centered care in clinical settings around the world. In 2008, the institute started a seminar series, "*The Process of Defining Hearing.*" It was during this seminar that the idea of exploring how the experiences of people with hearing loss change over time was proposed. The institute created a *possible patient journey* based on the collaborative work of over 60 professionals around the world who have worked in the area of hearing healthcare.

In 2009, Vinaya Manchaiah was made aware of this patient journey idea when he was invited to attend an Ida Institute seminar. At this time, Berth Danermark served as a faculty member of the institute. Following the seminar, Vinaya, in close collaboration with the late Professor Dafydd Stephens, started working on further developing the patient journey model by researching perspectives of those with hearing loss. After a few initial studies, in 2013, Vinaya went on to develop his doctoral thesis in this area titled, "Evaluating the process of change: Studies on patient journey, hearing disability acceptance and stages-of-change" at the Swedish Institute for Disability Research (SIDR), Linköping University, Sweden.

Since then there have been a number of publications in this area from researchers around the world. It is this research that led us to believe that there is a need for a book that provides details of these studies and ideas in a more accessible way to students and professionals who have interest in hearing loss.

In this edited book, we are happy to put together writings of numerous outstanding scholars from various fields, including: audiology, sociology, psychology, anthropology, and epidemiology. Each scholar has significant clinical and research expertise and first-hand knowledge about experiences of people with hearing loss. Multiple approaches are taken from audiological, psychological, and sociological standpoints to provide multi-dimensional understanding about experiences of people with hearing loss.

This book is aimed at future (undergraduate and graduate students) and present healthcare professionals (e.g. general medicine, gerontology, nursing, otolaryngology, psychology, etc.) to enhance reading about chronic conditions. In addition, we anticipate that this book will also be useful for early career communication disorder and audiology students to bolster reading for audiological rehabilitation courses. This book should be useful not only to professionals, students, and academics, but all those who themselves have experiences of hearing loss and their significant others.

Vinaya Manchaiah and Berth Danermark

ACKNOWLEDGMENTS

We would like to acknowledge the enormous contributions of our teachers, students, colleagues, and perhaps even more importantly those with hearing loss, for helping us in the development of the ideas for this book.

Vinaya would specifically like to acknowledge his friends, colleagues, and teachers, including the late Dafydd Stephens, Ilmari Pyykkő, Rajalakshmi Krishna, Basavarajappa, Fei Zhao, Berth Danermark, Barry Freeman, Thomas Lunner, Gerhard Andersson, Jerker Rönnberg, and Kerstin Möller for inspiring him with enthusiasm and creativity, as well as for helping him develop as a researcher.

Berth specifically acknowledges his colleagues for the willingness to respond affirmatively to the invitation to participate in this volume.

The book chapter authors have made significant voluntary contributions without which this edited book would not exist. We are grateful to them for their involvement, including meeting tight deadlines and positively considering our comments during the editing process.

Special thanks to Ross Roeser, Professor at the University of Texas at Dallas and Editor of the *International Journal of Audiology*, for writing the foreword for this book. Thanks also to Dr. Ashley Dockens for editing, proofreading, and formatting, which greatly improved the readability of this book.

We would also like to acknowledge the many publishers for their copyright permission to adopt some materials (i.e. figures, tables, and some text) from previously published work. These include: Hindawi Publishing Corporation (Chapters 1 and 4); John Wiley & Sons, Inc. (Chapters 3 and 14); *Journal of the Academy of Rehabilitative Audiology* (Chapter 3); Linköping University Electronic Press (Chapters 3 and 4); PAGE Press (Chapter 3); *PLOS One* (Chapter 3); and Taylor & Francis Ltd. (Chapters 1, 2, and 4).

Last but not least we are indebted to our family for their tolerance and encouragement during the preparation of this book. Vinaya greatly appreciates his parents,

Manchaiah and Manjula, his beloved spouse, Kavya Spandhana, and his friends, including: Jayaprakash Eraiah, Srikanth Chundu, Pradeep Rajegowda, and Mamtha, for all their patience and help. Berth is happy to acknowledge his wife, Gunilla, for her support and understanding of the work that needs to be done in order to edit a book like this.

ABBREVIATIONS

ABR	Auditory Brainstem Response
AR	Adult Aural Rehabilitation
BAHA	Bone-Anchored Hearing Aids
BICS	Brief ICF Core Sets for Hearing Loss
CICS	Comprehensive Core Sets for Hearing Loss
CP	Communication Partner
ENT	Ear, Nose, and Throat
GP	General Practitioner
HBM	Health Behavior Change Models
HHIE	Hearing Handicap Inventory for the Elderly
HHP	Hearing Health Professionals
HHQ	Hearing Handicap Questionnaire
HLAA	Hearing Loss Association of America
HRQoL	Health-related Quality of Life
ICF	International Classification of Functioning, Disability and Health
LASA	Longitudinal Aging Study Amsterdam
NL-SH	Netherlands Longitudinal Study on Hearing
OAEs	Otoacoustic Emissions
PCAR	Person-Centered Audiological Rehabilitation
PCC	Person-Centered Care
PHL	Person with Hearing Loss
SIDR	Swedish Institute for Disability Research
TMC	Transtheoretical Model of Change
WHO	World Health Organization

1

INTRODUCTION

Experiences of people with hearing loss

Vinaya Manchaiah and Berth Danermark

The need for this book

Disability is a complex phenomenon, which needs to be studied and managed with a holistic perspective. Moreover, disability experienced by an individual due to a specific condition (e.g., hearing loss) may be diverse in its nature and impact. Such chronic conditions cannot be understood fully by measuring its intensity during clinical encounters and documenting the objective limitations that the condition imposes (DePoy and Gilson, 2011). Therefore, it is important to clarify why acquired hearing disability affects people in the manner that it does. However, this may require a multi-dimensional approach and a study of *lived experiences* could be important.

Aural rehabilitation is the core component of dealing with hearing loss. There are wide ranges of books (from introductory to advanced) available with the focus on aural rehabilitation. Generally, texts on aural rehabilitation have focused on specific aspects of rehabilitation (e.g., hearing aids, cochlear implants, counseling), although some textbooks have a more extended scope. In addition, almost all, including those with wider scope, are written with a focus on the clinician and what they need to learn in order to offer appropriate aural rehabilitation for persons with hearing loss (PHLs). There is growing literature on the *patient's view*, which considers the processes that PHLs experience before, during, and after rehabilitation. These can include physical, mental, and social changes they face as they progress with different phases of their journey through hearing loss. Some autobiographical works have provided some accounts of this dimension. However, the authors of this book are unaware of any comprehensive book that captures this internal and external process that the patients and their communication partners (CPs or significant others) experience during the course of their condition. Hence, this book will focus on lived experiences of PHLs.

This book provides understanding of the main phases PHL may experience. It highlights the factors that may facilitate or hinder their progress through the course of the condition in terms of help-seeking, adopting rehabilitation interventions, adherence to rehabilitation, and outcomes of rehabilitation. Considering the patient viewpoint of the journey may provide some insights to the way they accomplish problem solving (or not) to cope with or manage their condition.

This book is written without assuming previous knowledge about disability and hearing loss. Hence, it can serve as an introductory book for various healthcare professionals. In addition, as it presents some new perspectives it can be a useful resource for hearing healthcare professionals. All the authors have a broad range of experiences in terms of working with a PHL, and have done in-depth study about the aspects discussed in their chapters with inspiration drawn from real cases. By employing experiences from people with technical, medical, and social science backgrounds, we believe this book presents a comprehensive view of hearing loss and disability with a focus on the patient perspective.

Finally, it is important to highlight that the scope of this book is limited to adults with gradually acquired hearing loss. We would argue that information in this book is complementary to popular rehabilitative audiology books, including Alpiner and McCarthy (2000) and Montano and Spitzer (2013). The book entitled *Living with hearing difficulties: the process of enablement* by Stephens and Kramer (2009) is the only other book that has taken the perspective of patients/clients, as far as we are aware, although it focuses much on aural rehabilitation models. Hence, the current book that provides an understanding of the processes from the patient's perspective can be helpful for clinicians and students.

Layout and content of the book

This book has 14 chapters, which are written by experts from different parts of the world with varied professional backgrounds (audiology, psychology, sociology, anthropology, and epidemiology). The central theme of the book is to present and detail the patient journey model of the PHL. Earlier chapters focus on introducing the concept of patient journey, most of the mid-chapters expand on each phase of the journey with clear examples, and later chapters focus on implications. Due to the nature of the patient journey model and the aim of the author to write each chapter so that it can be read independently of the other chapters, there is some overlap across chapters. However, this information is complementary.

Chapter 2 provides a discussion about functioning and the International Classification of Functioning, Disability and Health (ICF). Chapters 3 and 4 present the journey model of the PHL and their CPs. In Chapters 5 through 12, the seven main phases of the journey of PHLs are described. Chapter 13 provides an overall illustration of the journey based on a longitudinal study of PHLs followed for over 15 years. Finally, Chapter 14 provides insights to implications and practical applications of the patient journey model.

Main elements highlighted in this book

To capture various internal and external factors that the PHL experiences through different phases of their journey, the chapters in this book will focus on the following aspects:

- *Functioning:* Referring to operating in a particular way to fulfill a task or purpose. This has two elements: activity (i.e., capacity) and participation (i.e., performance). It is difficult to distinguish between activity and participation. Aspects such as commitment, energy, freedom, control, and self-realization can also contribute to functioning.
- *Conversation (or communication):* The informal exchange of ideas by spoken words.
- *Emotions:* A natural instinctive state of mind deriving from one's circumstances, mood, or relationships with others.
- *External conditions of life:* Home, work, finances, and interpersonal relationships (family, friends, etc.).
- *Inner psychological state:* Commitment, energy, feelings, self-realization, self-esteem, freedom, security, and state of mind.
- *Mood:* Valuing intangible things (e.g., harmony, balance, joy).
- *Relationships:* The way in which two or more concepts, objects, or people are connected, or the state of being connected.
- *Self-image:* Self-esteem, self-acceptance, close relationships, and friendship.
- *Dialogism:* Meaning is created through interaction, in dialogue.
- *Social recognition:* To be recognized by others as a complete human being.
- *Stigmatization:* To set marks of infamy or disgrace upon a person.

Evidence based practice

Evidence based practice (EBP) is the conscientious use of current best evidence in making decisions about patient care. The goal of EBP is the integration of: (a) practitioners' knowledge and experiences; (b) scientific or research evidence; and (c) patient, client, and caregiver perspectives to provide high-quality services reflecting the interests, values, needs, and choices of the individuals served. It is common for academic literature to focus on research evidence and expert opinion. In this book, we include all three elements, but patient perspectives are highlighted.

Theoretical framework

Our understanding of phenomenon (e.g., impairment and disability) is underpinned by concepts and the relationships of concepts. The following three conceptual or theoretical frameworks form the foundations of the chapters in this book: *Stages of change model; person-centered audiological rehabilitation (PCAR); and biopsychosocial model*. However, the *life-adjustment model* is also discussed in Chapter 13 to form an overall discussion about the patient journey.

A conceptual model (e.g., International Classification of Functioning, Disability and Health – ICF) is madeup of the important concepts that are used to help understand or stimulate a subject the model represents. It provides insight into what should be included in analysis of the phenomenon. A theoretical framework is a more elaborated conceptual framework and, together with definitions and reference to relevant scholarly literature and existing theory, provides a frame of reference to explain and predict a particular phenomenon.

Stages of change model

The stages of change (also known as transtheoretical) model is based on the assumption that behavior change is mainly focused on an individual's readiness to make a change and is achieved via various stages. Prochaska and DiClemente (1982) originally developed this theory to explain how smokers were able to give up their smoking habits or addiction. Although different versions of this model have been proposed over the years, a four-stage model has been used most often to describe different stages of change. The four stages include: (1) *precontemplation* – not thinking seriously about changing a specific behavior and not interested in help (i.e., often in denial); (2) *contemplation* – aware of the consequences of the problem and spends time thinking about the problem; (3) *action* – taking active steps to change their behavior; and (4) *maintenance* – successfully avoiding any temptation to give up the change they have made. In some stages of change models, additional stages such as "*preparation*" (i.e., stage in between contemplation and action where people are making preparation to take action by seeking information) and "*relapse*" (i.e., failure to comply with the change made and return to old habit) have also been included. Overall, the stages of change model suggests that the individuals in later stages are most likely to help-seek, take up intervention, adhere to the intervention, and possibly to display successful outcomes.

This model forms the foundation of the patient journey model, hence detailed discussion can be found in Chapter 3 and other chapters refer to this model. The number of stages may vary from different articles related to the stages of change model. However, throughout this book we refer to three stages (i.e., before rehabilitation, during rehabilitation, and after rehabilitation) and seven phases (i.e., pre-awareness, awareness, movement, diagnostics, rehabilitation, self-evaluation, and resolution).

Person-centered audiological rehabilitation

Person-centered care (PCC) is used to refer to many different principles and activities, and there is no single agreed upon definition of the concept. This may be because PCC is still an emerging and evolving area. In addition, if care is to be person centered, then what it looks like will depend on the needs, circumstances, and preferences of the individual receiving care. For example, what is important to one person in their healthcare may be unnecessary, or even undesirable, to another. It may also change over time, as the individual's needs change. Hence, instead of offering a concise and limited definition, the Health Foundation (2014) has identified a framework that comprises four principles of PCC. These principles include: (1) affording people dignity, compassion, and respect; (2) offering coordinated care, support, or treatment; (3) offering personalized care, support, or treatment; and (4) supporting people to recognize and develop their own strengths and abilities to enable them to live an independent and fulfilling life. Overall, PCC refers to providing care that considers individual preferences, needs, and values, and actively involves the individual affected in decision making.

This PCC concept has become popular in healthcare including in hearing health, with the term person-centered audiological rehabilitation (PCAR). From the perspectives of PHL, it is suggested that PCAR has three dimensions (Grenness et al., 2014). These include: (1) the therapeutic relationship between clinician, patients, and their family members; (2) the players (audiologist and patient); and (3) clinical processes. In addition, individualized care is suggested to be an overarching theme that links each of these dimensions.

The three fundamental principles of the PCAR are: (1) goal of rehabilitation is to alleviate consequence of disability to the person, their communication partners, and to society in general; (2) rehabilitation is a process; (3) rehabilitation is a client-centered problem-solving process, which can be better termed as "enablement." Table 1.1 presents the process and elements involved in PCAR (Gagné, 1998).

As this book focuses on the internal and external processes the patients may experience at different phases during their condition, the elements discussed in this

TABLE 1.1 Process and elements involved in person-centered audiological rehabilitation

Stages	Elements of person-centered audiological rehabilitation
Before rehabilitation	• Recognize that there is a problem • Identify the problem • Analyze the situation and describe the problem
During rehabilitation	• Set objectives and define desired outcomes taking into account: the problem; the person with hearing loss; the communication partners; the context; and the environment • Identify possible outcomes • For each solution identified, analyze and evaluate the implications of choosing that solution • Select one (or more) acceptable solution • Implement the solution
After rehabilitation	• Evaluate the effect of applying the solution (i.e., the objectives) • Identify the factors that facilitated, or constituted an impediment to, the implementation of the solutions

book help uncover important concepts of PCAR. Hence, having this knowledge may help clinicians to understand the hearing loss by standing in the patient's shoes (i.e., looking at different perspectives).

Biopsychosocial model

The biopsychosocial model is a general model or approach that considers biological, psychological (which entails thoughts, emotions, and behaviors), and social (socio-economic, socio-environmental, and cultural) factors, which may all play a significant role in human functioning in the context of health, illness, and disease (Suls and Rothman, 2004). The biopsychosocial model integrates biomedical (focuses purely on biological or medical factors) and social models (focuses purely on external societal factors) of disability. Hence, this model has a synergetic effect in understanding complex interactions of various internal and external factors that determine human functioning and health. The World Health Organization's (WHO) International Classification of Functioning, Disability and Health, also known as ICF (World Health Organization, 2001), is based on the biopsychosocial model (discussed in detail in Chapter 2).

It is important to note that the process of disease changing the quality of life can be influenced by external and internal biological factors (e.g., how the disease may lead to impairment). It may also be affected by contextual factors (e.g., personality, mental status, passiveness, sense of coherence, communication partners, and how impairments, activity limitations, and participation restrictions result in quality of life changes). This model highlights the fact that there could still be activity limitations and participation restrictions even in the absence of impairment and vice versa. These limitations can be temporary (e.g., people with normal hearing experiencing difficulty hearing in a challenging listening environment such as a restaurant) or permanent (e.g., not knowing the exact medical or pathological cause although the person may have limitations and restrictions due to poor hearing). Hence, adopting such a model in defining hearing loss and its consequences would be multi-dimensional (e.g., measuring impairment through audiological investigations and perceived disability using self-reported measures). To some degree, this model may help understand why we have such a diverse and heterogeneous group of people with hearing loss. As this book considers internal personal and external social factors in explaining the journey of a PHL, the biopsychosocial model forms the foundation.

Hearing loss and its consequences

Hearing loss is one of the most frequent chronic conditions in older adults. The World Health Organization (2015) estimates suggest that 360 million (328 million adults and 32 million children) people worldwide have disabling hearing loss (i.e., loss greater than 40 dB in better hearing ear in adults). This constitutes to over 5 percent of the world's population. Approximately one-third of individuals over 65 years have disabling hearing loss as measured, although more people may experience self-reported hearing difficulties in various listening environments and situations.

Hearing loss may have physical, mental, emotional, and social consequences for the PHL. There could be a range of adverse consequences mainly related to communication difficulties, relationship problems, reduced social interaction, social isolation, decreased self-esteem, and symptoms of anxiety and depression (as a consequence of misrecognition in society). These consequences may also result in poor performance in education and career and may have wider consequences for society. Although most of the consequences because of this chronic condition are negative, some individuals have been able to identify and report some positive consequences (or experiences). PHLs report that they use hearing loss to their self-advantage (e.g., say they did not hear when they don't want to hear or focus), affinity towards those with disability, being able to focus on certain tasks as they have reduced disturbance from unwanted external sounds and so on. The positive experiences in PHL are related to acceptance and coping rather than celebrating hearing loss like in the Deaf population. Table 1.2 presents the frequently reported positive and negative consequences to PHLs because of their condition.

Communication partners (CPs) of PHLs have also reported various adverse consequences. They may experience communication problems, confusion, anger, frustration, embarrassment, social withdrawal, and relationship problems and so on because of their partner's hearing loss. The WHO recognizes the limitations and restrictions experienced by significant others of people with disability as a third-party disability. In addition, CPs have also been able to identify various positive experiences because of their partner's condition. These may include: personal development (e.g., development

TABLE 1.2 Consequences of hearing loss (adapted from Manchaiah and Stephens, 2013)

Negative	• Increased difficulty communicating
	• Reduced interpersonal interactions
	• Avoidance and withdrawal from social situations
	• Increased loneliness, anxiety, irritability, anger, and frustration
	• Psychological problems such as depression
	• Decreased self-esteem and self-efficacy
	• Resultant (or increased) relationship problems
	• Increased risk to personal safety
	• Reduced ability to appreciate music
	• Reduced job performance
	• Reduced activities of daily life
	• Poor health-related quality of life
Positive	• Reduced disturbances from unwanted noise
	• Development of communication strategies
	• Affinity to people with hearing impairment and other disabilities
	• Perceived self-development
	• Using hearing impairment to self-advantage

of patience and tolerance); improved communication skills; understanding and awareness of hearing problems and so on. There is much variation in the consequences and coping of CPs and some may require help and support in their own right.

The congruence between perspectives of PHL and CPs are important in managing hearing loss and for living well with hearing loss. For example, if both PHL and CPs have accepted the condition and make a commitment to deal with its consequences then this mutual process results in better adjustment and coping. This is because the adjustment process involved both functional and social elements with the main strategy as prioritization of needs. Both PHL and CPs may have their own journey through hearing loss (discussed more in Chapters 3 and 4). Hence, it is important to understand consequences of hearing loss for both the PHL and CPs. Moreover, efforts should be made to address consequences for each of them individually and also together.

Encounters, interactions, communications, and emotions

To fully understand the implications of a hearing loss, a person must acknowledge that encounters, and hence interactions, are one of the basic dynamics of society. Interactions involve communication, which generates emotions (Danermark, 1998). Emotions are of great significance to our well-being. Disturbed communication is by far the most commonly reported effect of hearing loss and many consequences of hearing loss are of an emotional character. For instance, fear of losing face is crucial in interaction. Shame is an important emotion and often connected to losing face. It is often hidden, misnamed, or avoided. However, if shame is acknowledged, it is discharged. In traditional audiological rehabilitation, the focus is on aural perception, visual perception, and speech but less on emotional problems, like shame and embarrassment. Such emotions have to be brought to the forefront in PCAR.

Understanding and describing hearing loss

Disability and impairment have been understood in a number of ways, with either narrow or wider criteria. In general, wider criteria or definitions have been used when studying disability from a social science perspective. Disability has also been studied, understood, and described via various models, in both practice and research. Some such models include: biomedical, social, biopsychosocial.

Consequences of hearing loss (see previous section) can be seen at different levels. From a biological perspective, hearing loss is likely due to impairment in the auditory system and may affect various psychoacoustic (i.e., perception of sound) dimensions of the sense of hearing. These may include:

1.   *Threshold sensitivity (i.e., auditory threshold):* minimum sound level required to produce sense of hearing.
2.   *Dynamic range:* Range between minimum auditory threshold and uncomfortable loudness levels.

3. *Frequency resolution:* Ability to discriminate different frequency sounds.
4. *Temporal resolution:* Smallest sound duration the human ear can detect.
5. *Binaural hearing (or hearing with two ears) advantage:* Localization of sounds and ability to discriminate speech in the background noise.

A pathology in the external, middle, or inner ear may result in one or more of these dimensions. For example, pathology in the external and/or middle ear (i.e., conductive hearing loss) may result in decreased auditory thresholds, whereas damage to the inner ear (i.e., sensorineural hearing loss) may affect almost all the five dimensions mentioned above. Moreover, there may be a combined effect (i.e., mixed hearing loss) resulting in a combination of adverse consequences in sound perception.

These psychoacoustic dimensions provide an estimation of hearing based on various clinical measures. However, perceptual experiences (i.e., subjective experiences) of PHLs may vary from person to person in ways that cannot be measured. The variation can be related to differences in the extent to which the psychoacoustic dimensions are affected. However, often even with the same or similar psychoacoustic dimensions, individuals may report different perceptual experiences. This is because the subjective perceptual experiences may be further influenced by various internal and external factors. These factors can be broadly classified into: biological (or pathophysiological), social, environmental, and individual categories. Table 1.3 summarizes the main factors in these external and internal factors.

The way hearing loss is understood and how its consequences are managed may depend on: (a) perspectives of PHLs, CPs, and hearing healthcare professionals (referred to as clinicians or practitioners); and (b) external and internal influencing

TABLE 1.3 Four dimensions of factors that may influence the perceptual experience of hearing loss (taken from Manchaiah and Stephens, 2013 and reprinted with permission from Taylor & Francis Ltd)

Biological (or pathophysiological)	*Social*
• Type of hearing loss	• Communication partners
• Degree of hearing loss	• Employment
• Genetic factors	• Socio-economic status
• Pathophysiology	• Culture
• Cognitive functions (e.g., working memory)	• Social norms
Environmental (i.e., mainly referring to physical and/or acoustic domain)	*Individual (also includes psychological)*
• Background noise	• Age
• Directions of speech and noise	• Sex
• Orientation in the space	• Personality
• Number of people in the communication situation	• Family history
• Acoustics of the communication situation (particularly reverberation)	• Acceptance of hearing loss
	• Mental toughness
	• Lifestyle

factors. PHLs and CPs may define hearing loss based on their subjective life experiences. PHLs may define their hearing loss in terms of their difficulties in communication and limitations in various life situations (e.g., telephone, television). CPs may define the hearing loss from their own perspectives considering how hearing loss has altered their life, their relationship, and how both PHL and CP roles may have changed as a consequences of hearing loss. However, clinicians may define hearing loss primarily based on results of clinical measurements (e.g., type and degree of hearing loss, underlying pathology, speech understanding abilities). It is important to recognize that all these perspectives are important as they highlight different aspects of hearing loss.

The interactions between influencing factors are also important in defining and explaining hearing loss and its consequences. For example, the same person with a particular degree of hearing loss may have various performance and experiences in audibility and speech perception in different listening environments (i.e., influence of environmental factors). In addition, people with similar audiological characteristics (e.g., degree or type of hearing loss) may display varying degrees of communication problems with possible influences of biological, social, and individual factors. Hence, considering the potential influencing factors and different perspectives are important in the management of consequences of hearing loss (see Figure 1.1). This wider perspective in understanding hearing disability goes well with the biopsychosocial model of disability. In more concrete terms, the WHO-ICF may be a more appropriate model in understanding the broader consequences of hearing loss.

Generally, audiological textbooks focus heavily on the clinician perspective of hearing loss and biological factors, although some aural rehabilitation texts discuss all four main areas of influencing factors. In this book, the aim is to discuss the perspective of the PHL and, to some degree, perspectives of CPs. Although all four

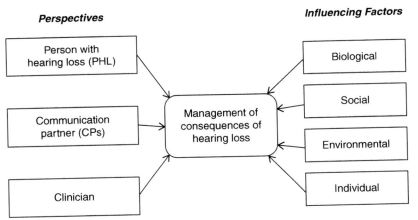

FIGURE 1.1 Perspectives and influencing factors that need to be considered while planning management of consequences of hearing loss (taken from Manchaiah and Stephens, 2013 and reprinted with permission from Taylor & Francis Ltd)

elements of influencing factors are discussed, there is less emphasis on biological factors and greater emphasis on social, environmental, and individual factors.

Longitudinal understanding of hearing loss

In recent years, there has been greater emphasis on measuring health outcomes in terms of function. For example, the WHO-ICF assumes interplay of factors at different levels (e.g., biological, psychological, social) and advocates understanding of disability in terms of impairment, ability, activity limitations, and participation restrictions (World Health Organization, 2001). In practice, the impairment is usually measured using clinical evaluations (i.e., subjective evaluation measured objectively), while disability (i.e., activity limitations and participation restrictions) is measured using self-reported outcome measures (i.e., subjective measures). Both impairment and disability may change over time. Measuring outcomes at different time intervals may provide better understanding of change over time. However, outcome measures are specific to some aspects and may not capture how the experiences of people with disability or a particular health condition change over time. Therefore, it is important to evaluate the process of change (i.e., process evaluation), because it could provide in-depth knowledge about mechanisms behind changes. In this book, *process evaluation* has been used in the context of understanding and monitoring the change longitudinally (e.g., several days to several years; Manchaiah et al., 2014).

Outcome measurement versus process evaluation

It is quite common to study and evaluate change when it comes to health and interventions. Outcome measures are tools used in assessing the change over time. However, in healthcare practice they are mainly used as a baseline measurement during initial consultation with the patient and after intervention. The change in the outcome measures is usually assumed to be due to the treatment or interventions. This is the typical design used in research trials with the classical OXO (one-group-pre-post) model. Outcome measures can have various purposes. For example: (a) to measure rehabilitative outcomes of an individual person with disability; (b) to assess the effectiveness of the service provided by a particular clinical unit or agency; (c) to assess the effectiveness of new technologies and treatment methods; and (d) to assess the effectiveness of rehabilitation services on quality of life (Cox et al., 2000). In addition, outcome measures have also been used to formulate intervention strategies. While outcome measures can be used longitudinally to measure change over time, they are primarily used just before and after treatment (Manchaiah et al., 2014).

Outcome measures provide information about a specific aspect (e.g., depression, anxiety, level of hearing disability, etc.) depending on the measures we are using and the extent to which the person is affected at that point of time. The Hearing Handicap Questionnaire (HHQ) is used to measure the psychosocial aspects of hearing disability, and is a good example of an outcome measure. Changes in outcome measures can also be used to evaluate the degree of success of an intervention. For example, with HHQ, lower perceived hearing disability after audiological management (e.g., hearing aids) suggests the benefits of the management approach used.

The process evaluation refers to studying the experiences of the person with disability in the form of a timeline to understand the main phases or stages they experience during a disease and treatment. Studies on the patient journey represent good examples of process evaluation. However, even though these studies on the patient journey uncover important information about the process of change in persons with disability and influencing factors, they may not capture the intensity to which the person is affected at a point of time. While there is some amount of theme identification in this, time is an additional dimension of this approach. In addition, it can be argued that the use of outcome measures at multiple intervals may act as process evaluation (i.e., continuous monitoring of outcomes using outcome measures). However, devising such a measurement tool to capture both outcome and process could be challenging.

In general, the practice of healthcare and disability management is dominated by the use of outcome measures. In a recent study focusing on the development of ICF core sets for hearing loss, it was found that there are over 100 different outcome measures in the literature related to adults with hearing loss (Granberg et al., 2014). It was also highlighted that there are very few longitudinal studies in relation to adults with hearing loss. Although the value of outcome measures is not in question, there seems to be little focus on understanding the process of change over time in relation to health and disability, which may highlight the need for studies on the patient journey of PHLs and their CPs.

Importance of process evaluation

While the use of outcome measures is common, it can be argued that both outcome measurement and process evaluation are important. Some inspiration for process evaluation can be drawn from the area of marketing and business studies. For example, the concept of a *product life cycle* refers to the stages that product or its category passes through, including: introduction to the market, growth, maturity, and decline. This model provides important information about the product over time. However, it is important to note that length of each cycle in each product varies greatly, and it may be impossible to know with certainty when a product moves from one stage to another. Despite these shortcomings, this model is still very popular in the area of marketing and business management in formulating strategy.

To better understand the difference between process evaluation and outcome measurement, let us consider a simple scenario where a person is travelling from place A to place B. His or her main goal in this context is to reach B. In this example, if you use only outcome measurements we can capture whether or not a person reached place B. It can include more variables (e.g., within a given time limit or using a particular route), but it does not capture the experience through this journey and how they changed over time. More importantly, what sort of factors may have positively or negatively influenced the journey? Even though most people may consider reaching place B a success, some may decide not to undertake that journey again because of difficult experiences they had through this journey or the opposite. This example suggests that the process evaluation may highlight various factors that cannot be fully understood through outcome measures. This way of thinking can be applied to a particular health condition and disability.

It is important to note that there are benefits and shortcomings of both outcome measurement and process evaluation. A discussion paper by Mant (2001) compares process and outcome measures as performance indicators in healthcare and suggested that healthcare is only one determinant of health, and other factors (e.g., nutrition, environment, lifestyle, etc.) may influence health outcomes. The differences in outcomes (measured with outcome measures and reflecting a wide range of aspects) may be due to various reasons (e.g., the types of cases for which the treatment was administered, how data was collected, chance, quality of care given, etc.). However, process evaluation could have some advantages as they are more sensitive to difference in quality of care and may act as a direct measure of quality. Mant (2001) also argued that the outcome measures are of use only where outcome indicators have the power to detect variation in healthcare leading to changes in health outcome and such changes are sufficiently common to produce enough power in outcome measures. For this reason, if these conditions are not met then other approaches (e.g., process measurement and risk management of individual incidents) could be more effective. Even though the perspectives expressed here are based on considering healthcare practice as a whole and discussing the strengths and weaknesses of outcome and process measures as healthcare performance indicators, the findings and recommendations have some use to each individual.

Overall, it is noteworthy that even though the approaches discussed above provide similar information, they give different perspectives in understanding the same condition. It can be argued that the combination of such approaches may give better understanding of a person with disability than any one approach alone. It is also important to establish a link between such combined approaches to better understand what information they are providing. Considering this, it is suggested that process evaluation is useful for disability research and may have clinical value.

Process evaluation: examples from studies on hearing loss

It appears in recent years that studying the lived experiences of persons with disability is becoming popular. Moreover, perspectives and opinions of disabled people are being considered at different levels of policy making. Studies on the patient journey represent one way of capturing these lived experiences of persons with disability. In addition, such studies also explore the process of change by considering various experiences a person may have during the initial onset of the disease, realization, acceptance, help-seeking, assessment, rehabilitation, and continued experience of a particular condition. Reported experiences can be analyzed to identify relevant

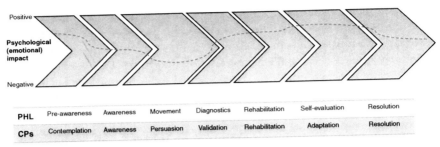

FIGURE 1.2 Journey of person with hearing loss and their communication partners. The various phases are not drawn to any scale in regard to duration, and time spent in each phase may vary between individuals (taken from Manchaiah et al., 2014 with permission from Hindawi Publishing Corporation)

themes and be represented in the way the themes reflect the data. Such an approach is often used in disability research while attempting to understand the lived experiences of a person. In a clinical setting, this is completed informally through case history.

The Ida Institute initially developed a model of the possible patient journey of PHLs and their CPs by considering the professionals' perspective. Studies have further developed these models by considering perspectives of PHLs (see Chapter 3) and their CPs (see Chapter 4). These models are illustrated in Figure 1.2, demonstrating the main phases experienced by PHLs and CPs from the initial onset of disease to diagnosis, treatment, and long-term living with the hearing loss. It is important to note that the various stages in the model are not drawn to any scale and the progression from one phase to another may vary from person to person quite considerably (i.e., several days to several years). This model does not measure the intensity at which PHLs and CPs are affected at any one stage or point. For this reason, outcome measures would be helpful in conjunction with this model to measure the intensity at which the person is affected at any point of time.

Studies on the patient journey of PHLs and CPs have considered hearing disability from a different dimension (i.e., temporal) and have provided new insights (Manchaiah and Stephens, 2011; Manchaiah et al., 2011; Manchaiah et al., 2013). Moreover, studies on the patient journey can also highlight some barriers to the help-seeking process that may not be identified through structured outcome measurements. For example, a study on the patient journey of sudden-onset hearing loss suggests that medical professionals did not always provide patients with the correct information about the condition and its expected prognosis (Manchaiah et al., 2012). This raises some general, ethical, and legal questions.

The phases represented in patient journey studies related to hearing loss appear to correlate well with the stages of change suggested in the *transtheoretical model of change*, which was proposed in relation to health behavior changes. This theory suggested that health behavior changes involve six main stages including: precontemplation,

contemplation, preparation, action, maintenance, and termination. This model is a cyclic or spiral model rather than linear which accounts for relapse and re-start. Such a model could be helpful while understanding the process of change through a disease (e.g., hearing loss) and its treatment.

How best to evaluate the process of change in a person with hearing disability?

Process evaluation can be studied and understood from perspectives of the person with disability, their significant others, clinicians, and in the wider context of society. However, it is important to note that priorities from each of these perspectives could be different. For example: (a) for people with disability and their significant others – their activity, participation, and quality of life could be key factors; (b) for clinicians – cure of impairment, reducing disability, and to some extent a quick fix to the problems reported could be important; and (c) for society – less dependency of people with disability on society and larger contributions from them could be important. Even though it is difficult to answer which of these perspectives is more important, considering the emphasis on *shared decision making* in recent years, the combined approach might be most helpful. Moreover, the process of change can also be evaluated from different analytical levels, which may include: biological, psychological, psychosocial, and socio-economic.

Studies on the journey of PHLs and their CPs have focused on an individual level by evaluating the reports of the PHL, their CPs, and clinicians. Moreover, these studies had relatively small sample sizes and employed research designs based on reported experiences, which may have been influenced by various aspects (e.g., perceptions and memory of the individuals). However, considering that the journey of PHLs and their CPs may take several years, longitudinal designs may be more appropriate. In addition, evaluating such models in a large population would be necessary.

Summary

Disability and impairment have been studied and understood from various models and perspectives. The most important point of departure from typical texts for this book is that hearing loss must be recognized as a lifelong process. In this book, this is described in terms of a journey, which highlights the importance of process evaluation and suggests that such an approach could make a significant contribution to better understanding disability (e.g., hearing loss). In order to fully grasp this journey we must highlight the human dynamics of hearing loss and include a number of perspectives and approaches. Special attention is paid to three such aspects: the stages of change model (i.e., the analytical division of the journey into seven phases), person-centered audiological rehabilitation, and the biopsychosocial model (illustrated by the WHO-ICF).

References

Alpiner, J. and McCarthy, P., 2000. *Rehabilitative audiology: children and adults*. 3rd ed. Baltimore, MD: Lippincott Williams and Wilkins.

Cox, R., Hyde, M., Gatehouse, S., et al., 2000. Optimal outcome measures, research priorities, and international cooperation. *Ear and Hearing*, 21(4), pp. 106S–115S.

Danermark, B., 1998. Hearing impairment, emotions and audiological rehabilitation: a sociological perspective. *Scandinavian Audiology*, 27(49), pp. 125–131.

DePoy, E. and Gilson, S., 2011. *Studying disability: multiple theories and responses*. California: Sage Publications, Inc.

Gagné, J.-P., 1998. Reflections on evaluative research in audiological rehabilitation. *Scandinavian Audiology*, 27(S49), pp. 69–79.

Granberg, S., Dahlström, J., Möller, C., Kähäri, K., and Danermark, B., 2014. The ICF core sets for hearing loss – researcher perspective. Part I: Systematic review of outcome measures identified in audiological research. *International Journal of Audiology*, 53(2), pp. 65–76.

Grenness, C., Hickson, L., Laplante-Lévesque, A., and Davidson, B., 2014. Patient-centred audiological rehabilitation: perspectives of older adults who own hearing aids. *International Journal of Audiology*, 53(S1), pp. 68S–75S.

Health Foundation, 2014. Person-centred care made simple: what everyone should know about person-centred care. *Health* [online]. Available at: www.health.org.uk/sites/default/files/PersonCentredCareMadeSimple.pdf [Accessed 16 March 2016].

Manchaiah, V. and Stephens, D., 2011. The patient journey: living with acquired hearing impairment. *Journal of the Academy of Rehabilitative Audiology*, 44, pp. 29–40.

Manchaiah, V. and Stephens, D., 2013. Perspectives in defining "hearing loss" and its consequences. *Hearing, Balance and Communication*, 11(1), pp. 6–16.

Manchaiah, V., Stephens, D., and Meredith, R., 2011. The patient journey of adults with hearing impairment: the patients' view. *Clinical Otology*, 36, pp. 227–234.

Manchaiah, V., Stephens, D., and Lunner, T., 2012. Information about the prognosis given to sudden-sensorineural hearing loss patients: implications to "patient journey" process. *Audiological Medicine*, 10, pp. 109–113.

Manchaiah, V., Stephens, D., and Lunner, T., 2013. Communication partners' journey through their partner's hearing impairment. *International Journal of Otolaryngology* [online]. Available at: www.ncbi.nlm.nih.gov/pubmed/23533422 [Accessed 16 March 2016].

Manchaiah, V., Danermark, B., Rönnberg, J., and Lunner, T., 2014. Importance of 'process evaluation' in audiological rehabilitation: examples from studies on hearing impairment. *International Journal of Otolaryngology*, Article ID 168684. http://dx.doi.org/10.1155/2014/168684.

Mant, J., 2001. Process versus outcome indicators in the assessment of quality of healthcare. *International Journal for Quality in Health Care*, 13(6), pp. 475–480.

Montano, J. and Spitzer, J., 2013. *Adult audiologic rehabilitation*. San Diego, CA: Plural Publishing.

Prochaska, J. and DiClemente, C., 1982. Transtheoretical theory: toward a more integrative model of change. *Psychotherapy: Theory, Research, & Practice*, 19(3), pp. 276–288.

Stephens, D. and Kramer, S., 2009. *Living with hearing difficulties: the process of enablement*. Chichester, West Sussex, UK: John Wiley & Sons, Ltd.

Suls, J. and Rothman, A., 2004. Evolution of the biopsychosocial model: prospects and challenges for health psychology. *Health Psychology*, 23(2), pp. 119–125.

World Health Organization, 2001. *International Classification of Functioning, Disability and Health (ICF)*. Geneva, Switzerland: World Health Organization.

World Health Organization, 2015. Deafness and hearing loss. *WHO* [online]. Available at www.who.int/mediacentre/factsheets/fs300/en/ [Accessed 16 March 2016].

2

FUNCTIONING IN ADULTS WITH HEARING LOSS

Sarah Granberg

Introduction

The notion of health is highly subjective. Some refer to physical aspects or conditions, such as whether one suffers from a disease or a disorder when discussing health; while some consider health, or absence of health, as connected to psychological or mental aspects or conditions often referred to as *well-being*. This ambiguity regarding the concept of health is also reflected in literature about the topic. Although the definition of health varies in different areas, it is common to view health from a biopsychosocial perspective in rehabilitation disciplines. This means that health is created through a complex interaction of biological, psychological, and socio-cultural factors. The concept of functioning is closely related to health. This is likely why the International Classification of Functioning, Disability and Health, ICF (World Health Organization, 2001) has ventured into the rehabilitation and health sciences in recent years. Based on biopsychosocial assumptions of health, the ICF has made a substantial contribution to the scientific and clinical rehabilitation work and literature.

Functioning and disability

Since the 1970s, the World Health Organization (WHO) has urged the evolution of classifications that focus on effects of health conditions or diagnosis when explaining and describing non-acute diseases. Several WHO classifications of this kind have been developed over the years. The last classification adopted, the ICF, is in use in clinical praxis or in research investigations. The ICF has embraced a health perspective where the concepts of functioning and disability are central. These concepts are made from the perspective of the body (anatomical and physiological aspects of body systems, organs and limbs including psychological functions), the person (a person's capacity to execute a task or an action, and a person's performance in the "real world" in relation to tasks or actions), and the environment (influential human-related or physical aspects in the environment). Human functioning is described with the positive concepts of body functions, body structures, activities, and participation; while disability is described with the negative terms of impairment (problems in body structures or functions), activity limitations, and participation restrictions. Of significant importance in the ICF is the non-causal relationship between the different concepts when experiencing disability. That is, impairment (such as hearing loss) does not automatically result in activity limitation or participation restrictions. Rather, it is the specific situation and the complex interaction between different aspects which result, in some cases, in disability. Consequently, functioning and disability in ICF is not a two-sided coin but rather a continuum where positive functional aspects can turn into disabling aspects depending on situational circumstances. A good example of this reasoning concerns persons who are culturally Deaf with sign language as primary communication mode. Deaf people have long claimed cultural status as a group and often prefer to be referred to as a minority group in society. For many persons, outside this particular group, Deafness is viewed as a major hearing disability because the individuals cannot hear. If one applies the underlying assumptions of functioning and disability in ICF in an example relevant for this group, the reasoning becomes clearer. Consider the following situation:

> Mr. Andersson went to the pub with Mr. Svensson. Mr. Svensson, like Mr. Andersson, is Deaf and uses sign language as his primary communication mode. They find a table in the crowded pub. However, they have to share the table with Mr. Hansson and Mr. Johansson. Mr. Hansson and Mr. Johansson have severe hearing losses and uses hearing aids. They are not part of the Deaf community and prefer oral speech as their primary mode of communication. The pub is extremely crowded and noisy today. Food and drink orders are shouted out behind the counter and people are just talking, laughing, and shouting everywhere. Mr. Andersson and Mr. Svensson have a blast! They have so many things to discuss, and so many observations to do! Mr. Johansson and Mr. Hansson, on the other hand, have a terrible evening. They cannot talk to each other because the noise is just overwhelming. They decide to leave, despite the early hour.

In the situation described above, one can certainly argue that while Mr. Andersson and Mr. Svensson had a wonderful evening and experienced no disability, Mr. Johansson and Mr. Hansson certainly did. In this case, conversation is central. Several aspects influence conversation in the above example. In the case of Mr. Andersson and Mr. Svensson, a probable profound hearing loss prevails for both of them and an important environmental factor would be the noise in the pub. However, both these aspects are irrelevant in this situation because the conversation is performed in sign language. They do not experience disability here. In the case of Mr. Hansson and Mr. Johansson, both have severe hearing losses and use hearing aids. In quieter circumstances, the hearing aids would help them to comprehend speech; however, in the present situation, these devices are not helpful at all. The environmental influence, in terms of noise, is so significant and overwhelming that it makes a substantial contribution to the experienced disability. The conclusion is that disability is always situational. Everyone can experience disability.

The International Classification of Functioning, Disability, and Health (ICF)

The conceptual model

Initially in the present chapter, the ICF was introduced and the theoretical assumptions underlying the classification were described. These theoretical assumptions can be disclosed in the conceptual ICF model (Figure 2.1). This model is widely spread and used in clinical practice, scientific literature, and in government policies.

At the top of the model is the label *health condition (disorder or disease)*. The ICF's original idea was to use it as a complement to medical/diagnostic classifications, to explain effects of medical disorders or diagnosis. A health condition in ICF could include diagnoses or disorders like hearing loss but also a circumstance such as pregnancy. Importantly, this is a model that identifies functioning, disability, and health of individuals with a health condition in specific situations; it does not label a certain group of people experiencing a certain health condition. The conceptual model has spread to be used outside the health care arena for assessing specific functional and health issues of people with no health conditions. In those cases, the label *health condition* has been disregarded and simply overlooked. This is acceptable

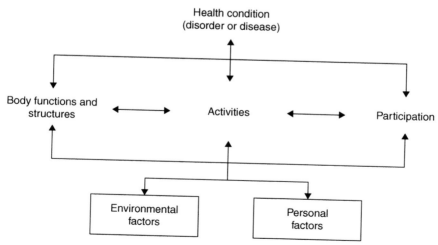

FIGURE 2.1 The conceptual model of the ICF (retrieved from World Health Organization, 2001)

because the label plays no actual role in the understanding of the model. It can therefore be ignored or simply replaced with "the person in front of me of whom I am assessing function and health."

In the center of the model (Figure 2.1) are activities. Activities in the ICF refer to a person's capacity to execute tasks or actions. In the area of audiology, an activity could be conversing with one person. If we consider this particular activity and try to imagine that it takes place in an office (such as the clinician's office), a person with a moderate hearing loss probably would manage reasonably well. If we instead "move" this specific activity out in the "real world" (e.g., to the street) what would then happen? In the ICF, this is referred to as *participation* (to the right in Figure 2.1) and assesses the "real life" performance of an activity. In this particular case, it is fair to argue that the performance is probably more difficult compared to what the person's capacity indicates because in the real world there are factors in the environment that influence performance. In the present area, such important factors could be noise or conversational behaviors of the person with whom you are conversing (the other person is covering his/her mouth or is turning away while speaking, etc.). The main difference between activity (capacity) and participation (performance) is, thus, that activities are executed without influence of the "real world" while participation is the actual performance experienced with influences of the environment. Many patients have concluded that several speech tests used in the area of audiology do not explain how it really works out for them in the "real world." This phenomenon could be explained with the ICF terminology. The speech tests that are used are primarily assessing body functions and capacity, and not aspects of performance. Currently, there are very few clinical tests, in the audiological field, that focus on performance (Granberg et al., 2014a). See Chapter 8 for discussion of this matter in detail.

To the left in Figure 2.1 are *body functions* and *body structures*. Body functions refer to the physiological functions (including psychological functions), whereas body structures are the anatomical parts of the body (e.g., organs, limbs). In audiology, it can be stated that hearing functions (body functions) are affected, to a varied degree, when one experiences hearing loss. The corresponding affected body structures could be the inner ear (cochlea) and the auditory nerve. In the example about conversing with one person, you can imagine that impairment in the hearing functions and in the corresponding structures would result in both worse capacity and a lower ability to perform in a conversation with one person, although to a varied degree. The performance is probably much worse than capacity. However, in the above example with Mr. Andersson and Mr. Svensson (who were Deaf and conversed in sign language), the impairments had no influence on the capacity or the performance to converse with one person.

At the bottom of Figure 2.1 are *environmental factors* and *personal factors*. Environmental factors are factors in the environment (human-related such as support or attitudes, or physical such as technology, design of public building, noise, or light) that influence the performance, either positively (acting as a facilitator to performance) or negatively (acting as a barrier to performance). In the example above about conversing with one person, environmental factors, such as noise and wind, are acting as barriers to performance. However, if we assume that the person has hearing aids, these would probably help in performance, acting as facilitators to conversing with one person.

Initially, in this section, it was explained that the starting point in the ICF model is the health condition of a person. In the ICF, there is an underlying assumption that there are certain human aspects (e.g., age or gender) that are not related to a person's health condition. These aspects are referred to as *personal factors* and can influence the performance. Returning to the example of conversing with one person, it can be assumed that aspects that are related to the natural aging process (e.g., overall physical health, cognitive aspects, and emotional state) could influence performance. However, personal factors in the ICF are difficult to handle and questions have been raised concerning whether aspects clearly related to the person (i.e., personal factors) can be truly separated from a person's health condition because the health condition is part of a person. Perhaps this theoretical issue will be solved and reflected upon in future updates of the classification.

ICF – a classification

The ICF is also a classification. Significant for a classification is the hierarchical structure and the labeling of different aspects in numerical codes. In the ICF, it is different aspects of human functioning (or health) that are classified with different numerical codes. Figure 2.2 illustrates the hierarchical structure in the ICF with provided examples relevant for audiology.

The ICF classification consists of two parts, Functioning/Disability and Contextual Factors. From each part, two components are derived: Functioning/Disability has the components of *body functions/body structures* and *activities/participation*, while contextual factors has components of *environmental factors* and *personal factors*. To each component, different categories are associated. The categories are organized in different levels (1st to 4th) where a category at a deeper level is a more detailed specification of a category on a previous level. Although body functions and body structures are viewed as one component, they have different associated categories (see Figure 2.2). Both body functions and body structures have eight chapters covering the different body systems. Activities and participation share categories. This is because, as discussed earlier in this chapter, an activity (capacity) is the dimension of a health category where the environment is not influential, while participation (performance) is the dimension of the same health category where the environment is influential. The health category is thereby the same; it is the way we assess the health category that determines whether a category is viewed as activities or participation. The different shared categories (sometimes referred to as health domains) intend to cover essential areas of human functioning. Examples of health domains are *communication; domestic life; interpersonal interactions and relationships; community, social, and civic life*. In total, nine domains (or chapters) are connected to activities and participation. The component of environmental factors has

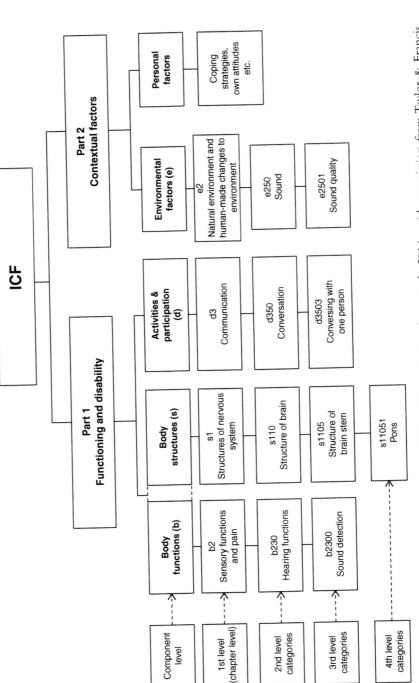

FIGURE 2.2 The hierarchical structure of the ICF (published in Granberg et al., 2014a with permission from Taylor & Francis. www.tandfonline.com)

five associated chapters. These chapters cover both the human-related environment, such as support or attitudes, and the physical environment, such as *products and technology* and *natural environment and human-made changes to environment*. The last chapter in the component of environmental factors is dedicated to *services, systems, and policies*. In the current version of the ICF, the personal factors component lacks categories. The reasons for this matter are various, but foremost cultural and international variations have been stated as main reasons for the non-classification of specific categories. This does not mean that personal factors are unimportant, on the contrary, it gives the person using the classification the freedom to classify whatever relevant personal factor he or she wants for each specific classified situation.

ICF Core Sets for Hearing Loss

Classifications are important when it comes to systematizing health conditions and the health aspects associated with them. Because the classifications are international, with a common language (the numerical codes), it allows a possibility to determine prevalence of health and illness. Furthermore, comparisons of different health aspects, both nationally and internationally, can be made and health care services and preventive actions can grow and develop. The WHO has also expressed that a very important use of the ICF is in clinical practice or in research investigations. Given that the classification is updated yearly with new health categories, the ICF contains about 1500 different categories. In reality, this means that if one wants to use the ICF, there are about 1500 categories to become aware of and of which to have knowledge. This specific matter serves as a huge barrier to clinical use of the ICF. The WHO has also acknowledged this problem and has therefore initiated the *ICF Core Sets project*. An ICF Core Set is a set of ICF categories (from different components) that are considered particularly relevant for a certain health condition, diagnosis, or situation. Therefore, when one wants to classify a health situation of an individual with a specific health condition, instead of choosing from 1500 categories, one can choose from about 120 categories. This is the case for clinicians or researchers in the field of audiology, at least the part of the field that deals with adults with hearing loss. In 2008, an initiative was taken by the Swedish Institute for Disability Research (SIDR) and the ICF Research Branch in close collaboration with many other international partners to develop the ICF Core Sets for Hearing Loss. At that time, no consensus was reached in the audiological field regarding the concept and meaning of *functioning*. This ambivalence was furthermore reflected in the great number, with different orientation, of self-assessment questionnaires that were used in the field to assess functioning.

The main idea when creating core sets is to develop two core sets, a *comprehensive*, and a *brief*. The comprehensive could be used in multi-professional settings, such as traditional clinical teams. The brief core set, which is derived from the comprehensive, could be used in single clinical encounters or in research investigations. The WHO has developed a rigorous three-phase, evidence-based procedure when developing core sets. This procedure was followed in the ICF Core Sets for Hearing

Loss project. In the first phase, the "evidence collecting phase", four scientific studies (preparatory studies) were carried out to investigate how the target group and professionals working with persons with hearing loss perceived functioning and health in adults with hearing loss. Furthermore, how these aspects are acknowledged in the audiological scientific literature, i.e., how scientists perceive functioning and health in adults with hearing loss, were also explored (Granberg et al., 2014a; Granberg et al., 2014b; Granberg et al., 2014c; Granberg et al., 2014d). All collected data was analyzed through the ICF to explain functioning and health from the ICF perspective. The results were thereby presented in specific ICF categories. In the second phase, a consensus conference, involving 21 experts (researchers, clinicians, and clients), was held to evaluate the evidence identified in phase one. The preparatory studies, with the specific ICF categories, were presented to the experts and they were instructed to carefully value and discuss the evidence. The outcome of this conference was the Comprehensive ICF Core Sets for Hearing Loss (CICS) and the Brief ICF Core Sets for Hearing Loss (BICS) (see Appendix section of this book). In the third phase, the two core sets should be assessed by field trials and other evaluations in order to determine their validity for the target group. The third phase is a currently ongoing phase. The two ICF Core Sets for Hearing Loss are published and available for use in clinical practice or in research investigations (Danermark et al., 2013).

Functioning in adults with hearing loss

The CICS contain 117 ICF categories and the BICS contain 27 categories. All ICF components are represented in both the core sets. In the BICS, only second-level categories are included. No categories that are not represented in the CICS are found in the BICS. In the CICS, 22 categories belong to body functions. Three body function chapters are covered in the CICS: Chapter 1 – Mental functions, Chapter 2 – Sensory functions and pain, and Chapter 3 –Voice and speech functions. Traditionally, audiology has focused foremost on the sensory auditory system, but in recent years, the importance of cognitive aspects in relation to hearing, listening, and comprehending speech have also been acknowledged. For example, research in the field has acknowledged the effort of listening, the impact of high cognitive ability when adjusting to hearing aids, and the reduced ability to shift and split attention to stimuli during conversations when having hearing loss (Pichora-Fuller, 2014; Rudner et al., 2009). These aspects are reflected in the core set and thereby recognized as relevant aspects of functioning. Emotional functions are also part of the core sets for hearing loss. In general, there seems to be an adverse relationship between aspects such as anxiety, depression, and feelings of loneliness and hearing loss (Gopinath et al., 2012; Nachtegaal et al., 2009; Pronk et al., 2011). This relationship can possibly be explained by the close relation between emotions and interactions (see Chapter 1 of this book). Maintenance of social bonds is crucial for social life. Threats of social bonds, which can occur when interaction is disrupted by hearing loss, can result in negative emotions. Emotions have been reported as the most significant outcome of interactions (Danermark, 1998). The consensus conference furthermore deemed the categories sensation of pain (b280) and energy level (b1300) as relevant for the CICS. In the preparatory studies, pain in the head and neck, were especially highlighted. Interventions targeting pain are usually not part of a traditional audiological rehabilitation approach but in some practices, physiotherapists are available for pain interventions. In addition, in recent years, complementary or alternative medicine techniques, such as yoga or mindfulness training, have made a foray into the traditional range of rehabilitation practices. For example, effects of yoga interventions have been scientifically evaluated in relation to health aspects such as stress and self-reported fatigue and are indicating promising positive results. Fatigue and decreased energy levels are problematic health aspects also in relation to hearing loss, and therefore, in the future, adults with hearing loss could be a suitable group for yoga trials or similar.

Concerning body structures, three chapters were identified as relevant, Chapter 1 – Structures of the nervous system, Chapter 2 – The eye, ear and related structures, and Chapter 7 – Structures related to movement. In the latter chapter, structures related to the head and neck region are particularly pointed out as relevant for the target group. In the audiological research area, the auditory system is viewed as one compound system starting at the outer ear, ending at the temporal lobe in the brain. This is not the case in the ICF, where the outer, middle, and inner ear are to be found in Chapter 2 while the auditory system beyond the inner ear (the central auditory system) is to be found in Chapter 1.

Many health aspects are considered relevant for the target group when it comes to the activities/participation component. Eight out of nine ICF chapters are covered in the CICS. It is very striking that many selected categories are relational. That is, the categories are not exclusively related to the person with hearing loss, but rather to the outcome of an interaction between two (or more) persons. Examples of such categories are conversing with one person or many people, discussion, interpersonal interactions, different relationships, school education, employment, and community life. Viewing these aspects in a rehabilitation perspective, the inclusion of significant others or other relevant communication partners (CPs) is essential when targeting these health aspects. This is very much in line with person–centered audiological rehabilitation (PCAR) where the collaboration between the affected person and his/her CPs is a necessary aspect in a rehabilitation program (Montano, 2014). Although several categories are relational, there are aspects that are clearly connected to the individual. For example, such aspects are watching, listening, receiving spoken messages (i.e., comprehending speech), handling stress and other psychological demands. The difference between hearing, listening, and comprehending speech is very important in the ICF because some of these aspects belong to different components. Kiessling and colleagues (2003, p. 30) provided useful definitions of the terms:

Hearing is a passive body function that provides access to the auditory world via the perception of sound. Listening is the process of hearing with intention and attention for purposeful activities demanding the expenditure of mental effort and comprehending speech is defined as the unidirectional reception of speech information, meaning and intent.

Although one can find the term "hearing" in many books, papers, or when people talk, it is quite often another level of auditory processing (i.e., listening or comprehending speech) that is referred to. This should be acknowledged, perhaps especially in rehabilitation settings, as it can help in guiding towards suitable rehabilitation interventions.

In the ICF, school education is not only targeting aspects such as gaining admission to school. In addition, the ability to engage in school-related responsibilities and working cooperatively with other students are relevant aspects of school education. The same reasoning applies to employment. Although having a job is essential, engaging in all aspects of work (e.g., seeking employment and getting a job; attending work on time as required; performing the acquired task alone or in groups; etc.) is also a highly relevant aspect of employment. The ICF thereby considers the role of being a student or an employee as vital when it comes to functioning and health. Former studies in audiology have highlighted essential aspects of being an employee or other issues related to employment associated with hearing loss. For example, such aspects are overrepresentation in early retirement, lack of control of work environment, and lack of control of work resulting in emotional distress (Fischer et al., 2014).

All five chapters in the component of *environmental factors* are represented in the core sets. Most categories from Chapter 1 – Products and technology covers assistive technological devices such as hearing aids, cochlear implants, and FM-systems but also regular technology that might have an impact on functioning have been highlighted. Examples of this are telephones, computers, and audio-recorders. A few categories targeting design and construction of both public and private buildings have been included. These categories include both technology that might have an influence on functioning such as loop-systems in public buildings, but also aspects related to acoustics, lights, etc. in public and private buildings. The human-related environment, social support and attitudes are viewed from the perspective of the individual. That is, how the individual experiences support and attitudes from others. Interestingly, hardly any research could be identified that focused on the human-related environment in the preparatory studies. In reality, this means that the vast majority of the research about environmental factors concerns technology, noise, or acoustics while social support or attitudes (both in close relations and in the society as such) are clearly neglected research areas. This result differed from the opinions of the target group and the professionals in the preparatory studies and at the consensus conference. The conclusion is that there seems to be an obvious discrepancy between the focus of research investigations compared to what the target group and professionals view as relevant environmental factors. This issue clearly has to be considered in future research investigations.

Summary

This chapter describes and explains the ICF and the key concepts of functioning and disability. The chapter also defines and discusses functioning in adults with hearing loss through the ICF Core Sets for Hearing Loss framework. Human functioning in ICF is described with positive concepts such as body functions and participation while disability is described with negative terms such as impairments and participation restrictions. Functioning and disability is viewed as a continuum where positive functional aspects can turn into disabling aspects depending on situational circumstances. Several functional aspects are relevant for adults with hearing loss such as memory, attention, and emotions. Many functional aspects are further relational and include interactions. This means that it is the outcome of the interaction that is important. Viewing this from a rehabilitation perspective, the focus must be on the person in his/her environment with relevant CPs. Furthermore, human support and attitudes are important for the target group. Unfortunately, many audiological research investigations concerning the environment focus on aspects such as technology and noise and thereby fail to acknowledge human support or attitudes. This matter needs to be further explored in future research investigations.

References

Danermark, B., 1998. Hearing impairment, emotions and audiological rehabilitation: a socio-logical perspective. *Scandinavian Audiology*, 27(S49), pp. 125–131.

Danermark, B., Granberg, S., Kramer, S., Selb, M., and Möller, C., 2013. The creation of a comprehensive and a brief core set for hearing loss using the International Classification of Functioning, Disability and Health. *American Journal of Audiology*, 22(2), pp. 323–328.

Fischer, M., Cruickshanks, K., Pinto, A., Klein, B., Klein, R., and Dalton, D., 2014. Hearing impairment and retirement. *Journal of the American Academy of Audiology*, 25(2), pp. 164–170.

Gopinath, B., Hickson, L., Schneider, J., et al., 2012. Hearing-impaired adults are at increased risk of experiencing emotional distress and social engagement restrictions five years later. *Age and Ageing*, 41(5), pp. 618–623.

Granberg, S., Dahlström, J., Möller, C., Kähäri, K., and Danermark, B., 2014a. The ICF Core Sets for hearing loss – researcher perspective. Part I: Systematic review of outcome measures identified in audiological research. *International Journal of Audiology*, 53(2), pp. 65–76.

Granberg, S., Möller, K., Skagerstrand, A., Möller, C., and Danermark, B., 2014b. The ICF Core Sets for hearing loss – researcher perspective. Part II: Linking outcome measures to the International Classification of Functioning, Disability and Health (ICF). *International Journal of Audiology*, 53(2), pp. 77–87.

Granberg, S., Pronk, M., Swanepoel, D.W., et al., 2014c. The ICF core sets for hearing loss project: functioning and disability from the patient perspective. *International Journal of Audiology*, 53(11), pp. 777–786.

Granberg, S., Swanepoel, D.W., Englund, U., Möller, C., and Danermark, B., 2014d. The ICF core sets for hearing loss project: international expert survey on functioning and disability of adults with hearing loss using the international classification of functioning, disability, and health (ICF). *International Journal of Audiology*, 53(8), pp. 497–506.

Kiessling, J., Pichora-Fuller, M., Gatehouse, S., et al., 2003. Candidature for and delivery of audiological services: special needs of older people. *International Journal of Audiology*, 42(s2), pp. 92–101.

Montano, J., 2014. Defining audiologic rehabilitation. In J. J. Montano and J. B. Spitzer (Eds.), *Adult audiologic rehabilitation*, 2nd ed., pp. 23–34. San Diego, CA: Plural Publishing, Inc.

Nachtegaal, J., Smit, J., Smits, C., Bezemer, P., van Beek, J., Festen, J., and Kramer, S., 2009. The association between hearing status and psychosocial health before the age of

70 years: results from an internet-based national survey on hearing. *Ear & Hearing*, 30(3), pp. 302–312.

Pichora-Fuller, K., 2014. Auditory and cognitive processing in audiologic rehabilitation. In J. J. Montano and J. B. Spitzer (Eds.), *Adult audiologic rehabilitation*, 2nd ed., pp. 517–534. San Diego, CA: Plural Publishing, Inc.

Pronk, M., Deeg, D., Smits, C., van Tilburg, T., Kuik, D., Festen, J., and Kramer, S., 2011. Prospective effects of hearing status on loneliness and depression in older persons: identification of subgroups. *International Journal of Audiology*, 50(12), pp. 887–896.

Rudner, M., Foo, C., Rönnberg, J., and Lunner, T., 2009. Cognition and aided speech recognition in noise: specific role for cognitive factors following nine-week experience with adjusted compression settings in hearing aids. *Scandinavian Journal of Psychology*, 50(5), pp. 405–418.

World Health Organization, 2001. *International Classification of Functioning, Disability and Health (ICF)*. Geneva, Switzerland: World Health Organization.

3

JOURNEY OF A PERSON WITH HEARING LOSS

Vinaya Manchaiah and Berth Danermark

Introduction

In this and the following chapter, the journey models of the person with hearing loss (PHL) (Chapter 3) and of the communication partners (CPs) (Chapter 4) are illustrated. Details are presented on each phase of the journey and examples are provided in the form of case studies.

Consequences of hearing loss

Hearing loss is a common chronic condition in middle-aged and elderly adults, which is often poorly recognized and rarely acknowledged. Acquired hearing loss can be caused by various sources, including genetic factors, noise exposure, ear disease, and others. Those with hearing loss may experience poor health-related quality of life due to consequences in both physical and mental domains (Chia et al., 2007).

A PHL may experience a variety of adverse consequences including communication difficulties, relationship problems, reduced social interaction, social isolation, decreased self-esteem, and symptoms of anxiety and depression. These consequences may also result in poor educational and vocational performance, and may have wider consequences to society. However, some PHLs have been able to report some positive experiences as a result of their condition. These include: using hearing loss to their self-advantage; developing affinity towards those with disability; being able to better focus on certain tasks; reduced disturbance from unwanted external sounds and so on. Moreover, hearing loss may also have adverse consequences to CPs of PHLs, which include spouse, children, relatives, friends, and colleagues.

Frequently, individuals may not be aware of the consequences they could face during this long journey of acquired hearing loss. However, they will have various experiences and milestones before, during, and after the hearing healthcare assessment and/or rehabilitation sessions (Manchaiah and Stephens, 2011). The natural course of the condition may vary and a wide range of long-term experiences have been reported by individuals with hearing loss (Edgett, 2002; Stephens and Kramer, 2009). Examples include: becoming aware of the problem; making a decision to seek help; achieving referral; and understanding hearing loss and its impact. This information may be invaluable to hearing healthcare professionals when they consider how best to ensure meeting the individual needs with treatment and/or rehabilitation options available.

Stages of change model

As indicated in Chapter 1, a stage of change model is a guiding principle for the outline of this book. Here we will further expand on this model generally before presenting the applications of this model within the context of hearing loss.

Health behavior change refers to facilitating alterations of habits or behavior related to health (Manchaiah, 2012). There are several proposed models that provide a theoretical framework for studying and understanding health behavior change. One example is the *transtheoretical model of change* (TMC; Prochaska and DiClemente, 1982). Although the transtheoretical model includes other concepts such as processes of change, decisional balance, self-efficacy, and temptation (Prochaska et al., 2009), in this book we focus on its stages of change aspect. The transtheoretical model is more popularly known as the stages of change model. It has been suggested that *health behavior change models* (HBMs) could be useful in audiology research and practice (Manchaiah, 2012).

The stages of change model was originally developed in the late 1970s and early 1980s by James Prochaska and Carlo DiClemente at the University of Rhode Island, while these researchers were studying how smokers were able to give up their habits or addiction (Prochaska and DiClemente, 1982). This model was utilized in health psychology, establishing that people go through various stages when they are trying to change behaviors (e.g., stop drinking, stop smoking, stop overeating). While researchers have proposed different versions, most often a four-stage model has been used to describe different stages of change. The four stages include: (1) *precontemplation* – not thinking seriously about changing a specific behavior and uninterested in help (i.e., denial); (2) *contemplation* – aware of the consequences of and spends time thinking about the problem; (3) *action* – taking active steps to change their behavior; and (4) *maintenance* – successfully avoiding any temptation to give up the change they have made. Some *stages of change models* also suggest additional stages, which include: *preparation* (i.e., a stage in between contemplation and action where people are making preparation to take action by seeking information); and *relapse*, after *maintenance* (i.e., failure to comply with the change made and return to old habit). According to the stages of change model, individuals in later stages are most likely to seek help, adopt intervention, adhere to the intervention, and possibly to display successful outcomes. In other words, the stages of change model focuses on an individual's readiness, with the assumption that the higher readiness results in greater possibility to make a change.

The stages of change model has also been applied in audiological rehabilitation. Currently three published studies have reported stages of change characteristics of adults with hearing loss in different stages and have identified four stages (i.e., pre-contemplation, contemplation, preparation, and action). Manchaiah and colleagues (2015) studied the stages of change characteristics in adults noticing hearing difficulties but who had not taken action. Laplante-Lévesque and colleagues (2015) reported stages of change characteristics in those who failed online hearing screening and also in adults with acquired hearing loss seeking help for the first time (Laplante-Lévesque et al., 2013).

With the stages of change model, it can be predicted that most individuals with hearing disability who see a clinician for help will be in the action stage (Laplante-Lévesque et al., 2013). Assuming that this model also has good predictive validity with people from the general population, it is reasonable to assume that the rest of the population with hearing disability who are not seeking hearing-help actively may be in pre-contemplation, contemplation, or preparation stages. If they are not aware of their hearing difficulties or are in denial, they are likely to be in the pre-contemplation stage. However, if they are aware of their difficulties but not actively seeking hearing-help, they are likely to be in either the contemplation or preparation stage. As Figure 3.1 exhibits, this pattern can be viewed in published studies on hearing loss. Nearly 90 percent of the people who are noticing hearing difficulties and taking online hearing screening are in the contemplation and preparation stages (Laplante-Lévesque et al., 2015; Manchaiah et al., 2015), whereas nearly 80 percent of those making first consultation with audiologists are in the action stage (Laplante-Lévesque et al., 2013). Although much work needs to be done in hearing healthcare to explore stages of change characteristics of PHLs, thus far results have been promising, supporting the applications of the stages of change model. However, based on observations, researchers suggest that change might be better represented on a

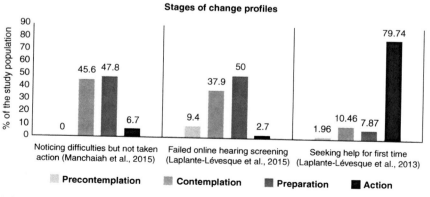

FIGURE 3.1 Stages of change profiles of people with hearing loss

continuum rather than movement in discrete steps (Laplante-Lévesque et al., 2013; Manchaiah et al., 2015).

Of note, research in this area has mainly focused on the early stages (i.e., becoming suspicious, seeking information, or seeking help) of the hearing help-seeking journey and not much is known from this theoretical perspective on later stages of the journey (i.e., acceptance of rehabilitation, adherence to treatment/management, successful or not successful use of rehabilitation).

Patient journey through hearing loss

The term *patient journey* refers to understanding the experiences and the processes that the patient experiences during the course of a disease and its treatment regime. It is believed that understanding this patient journey can help clinicians gain insight into the unique experiences of patients. In the last decade, with increased focus on patient-centered treatment approaches in healthcare, studies of the patient journey have become more popular.

Even though the onset of the disease may differ, the process and the stages experienced by the majority of patients are assumed to be broadly similar. Some information about the patient journey can be obtained while taking the case history. However, such information is often very limited due to time constraints. In addition, the content of the interview is generally led by the clinician rather than by the patient. It is very important for healthcare providers to understand and distinguish between illness (i.e., how the patients, family members, and the wider society view problems) and disease (i.e., how the healthcare providers view patient problems). Hence, the World Health Organization (WHO) advocates patient empowerment based on research from theories of stages of change and decision balance in order to facilitate the process of change (World Health Organization, 2012).

Furthermore, medical anthropologists have studied the course of illnesses related to various chronic conditions. Examples of published case studies with emphasis on the patient journey have been reported in a number of medical conditions, including: Parkinson's disease, Locked-in syndrome, Pertussis (whooping cough), and Rheumatoid arthritis. The clinical healthcare literature usually focuses on technical and physiological aspects of chronic disease management. However, some studies by anthropologists have focused on understanding the social and cultural dimensions of the illness. In recent years some healthcare professionals have attempted to better understand this process, which may assist in the development of a patient-centered treatment approach. For example, Edgett (2002) highlighted the process of making decisions to seek hearing help. This included four main stages: (1) understanding hearing loss; (2) personal experiences; (3) interaction with society; and (4) taking action. Also, Engelund (2006) studied the decision-making process of hearing impaired people who seek help, a process which she termed the "time for hearing." She identified four main stages experienced by patients during this process, which include: (1) attracting attention; (2) becoming suspicious; (3) sensing tribulation; and (4) jeopardising fundamental self. These studies provide some understanding of the typical process involved in hearing help-seeking although the later part of the journey was not emphasized.

The Ida Institute has developed a possible journey model for PHLs in collaboration with the efforts of hearing healthcare professionals around the world, which includes six stages: (1) Pre-awareness; (2) Awareness; (3) Movement; (4) Diagnostics; (5) Rehabilitation; and (6) Post-clinical (Ida Institute, 2009). Studies in medical anthropology reflect variations in the perspectives of the patients and professionals that may be due to differences in educational, ethnic, and socioeconomic backgrounds (Hunt and Arar, 2000). These variances in opinion and perspectives can have important implications for the effective management of a chronic condition. Understanding such differences may help healthcare providers to achieve a better appreciation of their patients' viewpoints. For this reason, it is important to explore the patients' perspectives of the journey.

The patients' view was added to further develop the *patient journey model*, and a new phase "self-evaluation" emerged. Hence, the updated patient journey model has seven main phases: (1) Pre-awareness; (2) Awareness; (3) Movement; (4) Diagnostics; (5) Rehabilitation; (6) Self-evaluation; and (7) Resolution (Manchaiah and Stephens, 2011; Manchaiah et al., 2011). Although some differences among professionals' and patients' view of the journey exist, they have much in common. Figure 3.2 shows the phases of the *patient journey model* of PHLs. This model represents the typical journey in adults with gradual onset hearing loss. However, those with sudden onset hearing loss may have a similar journey although often the pre-awareness phase is missing and they progress through the early phases of the journey (i.e., awareness to diagnostics) more rapidly (Manchaiah and Stephens, 2012).

It is important to recognize that the patient journey may not be linear; rather there may be some cyclic movement back and forth between different phases as indicated in Figure 3.2. It is illustrated in Chapter 13 that time spent in each phase may vary markedly from person to person (i.e., several days to several years) and there may often be some overlap in some phases. For example, a person may be becoming aware of the difficulties and have accepted hearing loss (i.e., awareness) and at the same time they may be seeking information and making decisions to seek help (i.e., movement). It is almost impossible to precisely identify which phase the person may be at one point in time. However, with clinical questioning, the clinician may be able to gain clear understanding of the likely phase the PHL may be in. Hence, considering the change as a continuum rather than movement in

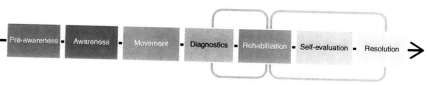

FIGURE 3.2 Main phases of patient's journey through their hearing loss (adapted from Manchaiah et al., 2011 with permission from John Wiley & Sons, Inc.)

discrete steps as suggested by some researchers may have some advantages (Laplante-Lévesque et al., 2013; Manchaiah et al., 2015).

As clearly illustrated by Laplante-Lévesque and colleagues (2012), "participants rarely described clinical encounters towards hearing help-seeking and rehabilitation as a connected process. They portrayed interactions with clinicians as isolated events rather than chronologically-ordered steps spanning over time and relating to a common goal" (p. 102). It is an important point to consider that PHLs may or may not see hearing help-seeking and rehabilitation as a series of isolated events, hence they may be unaware of the steps involved in hearing help-seeking and rehabilitation (see Chapter 13). However, in patient journey studies many participants reported their experiences in chronological order, similar to a timeline, even though they had gone back and forth when describing the experiences. This may be to some degree related to their memory. Nonetheless, when the patient journey model was presented to PHLs they were generally in agreement with the template as an accurate model representing their experiences (Manchaiah et al., 2011). Hence, the idea of the patient journey model can be useful when conceptualizing the change of experiences for PHLs over time.

We have in this book attempted to discuss each of the seven phases in order to enhance understanding of living with hearing loss. Chapters 6 through 12 will present in-depth discussions about each of these phases. However, it is important to note that there is limited literature on pre-awareness (in Chapter 5) and self-evaluation (Chapter 10) phases of the PHL journey. There is also a need for further research of PHLs' experiences and coping strategies in these phases. In discussion of these phases, both PHL experiences and professional experiences of the authors, including case studies, are used to provide a comprehensive view of the patient journey.

1. Pre-awareness

In this phase, the patient indicates their experiences before they become truly aware of their problems. The patients may show avoidance behaviors, but their family and friends may become increasingly aware of hearing difficulties, noting changed behaviors of the PHL (e.g., talking too loud). However, the PHL may be managing problems caused by the hearing loss without realizing the source of the difficulty. In addition, they often face uncomfortable and/or challenging situations in communication. This may cause feelings of frustration and bewilderment in PHLs and they may also notice such behaviors in their CPs.

2. Awareness

The person may start to become aware of their hearing loss following various specific experiences. In this phase they may also begin to notice other symptoms (e.g., tinnitus). The PHL begins to realize their problems and tries to map difficulties via self-testing in various ways (e.g., varying the TV volume or listening to various environmental sounds to test audibility).

3. Movement

After becoming aware of the problem and going through various experiences, the person may choose to do something about the problem. This could include obtaining input from their general practitioner, friends, media, and web. The PHL could then make a decision to seek help and arrange referral to a hearing healthcare professional.

4. Diagnostics

This is a phase that may be regarded as an active phase by hearing healthcare professionals. However, related aspects identified by patients include: difficulty experienced by PHLs in communicating problems to the clinician, undergoing hearing tests, and considering recommendations from hearing healthcare professionals.

5. Rehabilitation

In this phase, PHLs were able to identify many aspects including: obtaining treatment and hearing aid fitting, gaining access to assistive technology such as telephone amplifiers and FM systems, attending lip reading classes, learning and performing general maintenance of hearing aids, completing modifications to hearing aids (mainly in terms of gain) during audiological review sessions, and trying hearing aids from other hearing healthcare providers.

6. Self-evaluation

This is a new phase, which was identified only by patients. It includes: trying to assign reasons for their hearing loss; understanding the problem in terms of percentage of hearing loss; reflecting on positive and negative aspects of hearing aids in various situations; accepting or rejecting hearing aid(s); and evaluating the treatment received from different places.

7. Resolution

This phase was titled as post-clinical in the Ida template (Ida Institute, 2009) to refer to similar stages or milestones described. However, we believe that it may only describe the time of occurrence, not the content of the phase. For this reason, the term *resolution* is used, to best describe the following: the PHL undergoing adaptation and change, considering social impact, considering cost and time, having problems satisfactorily resolved or not resolved, and identifying new problems.

Case examples

The following life stories describe the impact of hearing loss on the PHL's life (Manchaiah and Stephens, 2011). The main issues pointed out by these individuals have been described in the seven main phases briefly described above (Manchaiah et al., 2011).

Jenny's story

Jenny is a 59-year-old female who has bilateral bone-anchored hearing aids (BAHA). She has retired and lives in South Wales. She first experienced hearing loss when she was a little girl (approximately 5–6 years old). This was caused by chronic ear infections and she underwent several ear operations (mastoidectomies) during her childhood. Having to take a lot of time off from school to go for treatment caused many problems with her education. Jenny reports that she had a very understanding family who supported her well during her childhood. She discontinued school at the age of 15 years and became a hairdresser. She has travelled widely and also worked abroad. Her ear infections continued and she suffered further difficulty with her hearing. However, because of constant active ear infections, she was not able to use hearing aids.

Jenny was advised that she would be a good candidate for bone BAHAs when she was in her early 30s. It was not until ten years later that she was implanted. The BAHAs helped her hear better and made a significant difference to her quality of life. Even with considerable problems hearing customers, she managed to keep her job until her early 50s. Jenny has faced a number of challenges due to her hearing loss. The following sections provide insight into some of the key phases and experiences through her journey with hearing loss.

Pre-awareness and awareness

Jenny was born and grew-up in the South Wales Valleys. She remembers her childhood with many ear operations as a distressing time.

> When I was a child I had lots and lots of mastoid operations. I used to scream in pain.

The nurse who attended the school for regular health checks first identified that she might have a hearing loss. Jenny's words describe the problems she faced during the initial stages of hearing loss. She notes her sense of separation and isolation from peers impacted on her education.

> Your schooling becomes affected, because you have taken so much time off to go for these operations. Even though they educated us in the school … you don't make the contact with the school-friends. Because by the time you

gone back to school they have either gone better ... your schooling does become affected ... Even though I think I could have done better as I went on to do other things and my education came when I went to work ... I learnt more when I left school than when I ever did in school.

There was hearing loss in Jenny's family. Her mother and her brother both had similar problems. She feels that, because of this, they were able to better understand the problems she faced and therefore supported her. She reports that communicating when at home was not a big problem as they all spoke to each other loudly.

TV and radios were always loud at my home. My mother and brother had hearing problems and we spoke very loudly ... we were a loud family.

Movement

The problems in communication continued and caused her more difficulties when Jenny became a hairdresser. She also needed to take time off to visit the doctors regularly while undergoing ear surgery, which created problems with employment.

When I started my job as a hairdresser, there were things I used to get wrong what people have said. I was not wearing hearing aids. I found it very difficult.

She mainly relied on information from the doctors about her ear disease and the treatment options.

Diagnostics

Jenny mainly visited otolaryngology (ear, nose, and throat [ENT]) specialists for treatment of her ear infections. However, she also had hearing tests routinely. She was not able to use traditional hearing aids because of her ear infections. Eventually, one of the ENT specialists recommended a BAHA for her.

When I found out about this bone-anchored hearing aids, I wanted one ... I heard about the BAHA from this American doctor in London.

Rehabilitation

Regular attendance to a hearing clinic has been a constant feature throughout Jenny's life. In the initial stages, she mainly sought medical help from hearing healthcare professionals.

Up until 30, I had about four ear operations.

However, she has been using BAHAs since she was in her late 30s.

> My hearing went right down. I went to see ENT. He was trying to get me to wear hearing aids. I couldn't wear the hearing aids due to infections. I was having recurring ear infections. I was deaf.
>
> I waited for about 10 years before having BAHAs … when I came to Wales. I kept saying about it. When the funding came through. There was a nice lady who showed the video. I really didn't care. I felt this is the way forward for my life.

Having a BAHA implanted was a major transition in Jenny's journey. She reports that she is doing well with the BAHA and manages well in most situations.

> This is one of the best things that has happened to me in my life.

Self-evaluation

Jenny reported having missed all sorts of sounds when she was not able to use any amplification devices because of ear infections. She understood what she was missing only after she started using the BAHA.

> I never heard water running through pipes for long time … rain … rain on the windows I never heard unless it is very, very loud.

While Jenny had experienced various difficulties in communication at school and work, her emphasis during the interview was on the emotional disturbances she experienced, mainly due to people not understanding her difficulties. A sense of stigma was also evident.

> People tend to think you are daft when you don't hear well.

Even though the hearing loss caused various challenges in physical and emotional terms, she was able to identify some positive aspects of hearing loss.

> I travelled a lot because of deafness and … because of my hearing I became more visual and I got better at my job. I was used to watching people … people watching … and get things right by watching and guessing … I also bluffed a lot … it also made me more determined and I think it did make me stronger. By travelling … you meet different people and nobody knew about my hard of hearing and I got by better.

Resolution

The life adjustment Jenny has had to make due to hearing loss has resulted in a poor quality of life.

It affected my job and affected my self-confidence. Luckily, I kept my self-confidence keep going until my last job … it did get me down so much that I suffered from depression.

People not understanding the hearing loss was very frustrating.

Oh … don't worry … she is deaf … you look back, you look at that and think … hang on … I am not able to hear so much, but there are ways in which they need to be educated not me …

Hearing loss can also act as a barrier when it comes to relationships and making friends.

People been saying to me I called you the other day and you ignored me … You can lose friends unless they can understand … you can lose people … you know … that you would like … but they think you are rude … because you have not heard … Deafness is an unseen disability … you don't carry anything to say you have it.

The other important issue identified was that people with acquired hearing loss might not have an easy access to support networks.

But maybe when you get deaf when you are young … you have a network, you learn sign language … I am not saying it's a lucky thing … but when you're caught in the middle and can't wear hearing aids due to infections … it saps your confidence so much … you feel like a non-person.

Having faced the hearing loss most of her life, Jenny had several comments and recommendations which need serious consideration.

I think what needs to happen is that … there needs to be somewhere where people can go and have support and counseling, not just for them and for the family, so they can handle it and through the family handling it, the society can handle it.

Alan's story

Alan is an 83-year-old man who developed hearing loss as he became older. He started noticing hearing difficulties when he was in his early 60s. He initially complained that his family members were mumbling and managed hearing loss for a few years without any help. However, due to family pressure, and also with the increase in the amount of difficulty he was facing, Alan consulted hearing healthcare professionals. He has been using hearing aids since he was in his early 70s. Alan notes that he manages well with his hearing aids in quiet situations, but finds it challenging to hear in situations with background noise present (e.g., restaurants, supermarkets). He is dependent on his wife, to some extent, for communicating in challenging situations, especially when using the telephone.

Pre-awareness

During the initial days of facing hearing difficulties, Alan expressed denial and blamed his family for not speaking clearly. However, with repeated complaints from family members he began to become aware of his hearing loss.

> First of all ... my wife and my children ... who said ... you are getting deaf. We are not mumbling ... you can't hear us. It's your fault.

Awareness

Alan reported that he started going deaf in his 60s. His hearing loss was confirmed when he had a hearing test.

> Specialists come and tested me at home ... commercial. Exactly when and what happened ... I am not sure. They said ... yes ... you needed a hearing aid. They fitted me with one.

Movement and diagnostics

Alan was first tested and fitted with hearing aids by a private hearing aid dispenser. He does not remember whether he consulted any other services. However, later he was referred from his family doctor to visit the Audiology clinic in the National Health Service, United Kingdom. He received services from them ever since.

> Later ... after a few years. In 1993, I must have gone to Singleton Hospital. Because, I have a book with the record. They tested me and I started getting National Health hearing aids.

Rehabilitation

He started noticing immediate benefits from hearing aids.

> I went home and I said to my wife, I have been hearing better than I have heard for years.

Alan is very dependent on his hearing aids.

> If I switch my hearing aid off ... I can't really say what you are saying ... I can't lip read either. I am in trouble.

Self-evaluation

Alan wears his hearing aids all day and finds it hard to manage without them.

> Sometime I can't understand my wife, particularly in bed at night … she speaks and I have to go face to face and watch her mouth. I can't lip read … but it helps.

Alan avoids conversations with visitors, especially if they speak quickly or have a strong accent.

> If we have visitors very often I sit back and I let them talk. I can't follow conversation.

He reported the following positive and negative experiences with hearing loss.

> The main positive experience is that it's quite nice to switch them off and listen to the silence. It's peaceful. It can be … but the real trouble is of course I might miss hearing things and I can't follow … Particularly if we are visiting someone or travelling or something … I miss picking up pieces of information … I do rely on my wife.

Resolution

Alan reported having difficulty with television and films.

> Films … I often can't follow dialogue, in TV. I can usually follow the news-readers … they are nice and clear … otherwise … in plays and so on … and quiz, shows, and so on … I have to use text at the bottom to follow what is happening.

He also experiences difficulty understanding people in challenging situations.

> If I go into a shop I can't always say what the shopkeeper is saying … particularly if there's other noise in the shop … my wife is an interpreter for me.

When questioned directly, Alan thinks that hearing loss did not interfere with his quality of life. However, during the interview several statements he made clearly identify the life adjustments and compromises he has had to make. Also, he identified the fact that hearing loss is not easily recognized and/or acknowledged by other people.

> If you are blind you have a white stick and they know you are blind. But when you are being deaf … unless you have a little sign saying "I am deaf" … they don't do anything about it.

Applications of the patient journey model

In an era where healthcare is driven by evidence-based practice and service user satisfaction, better understanding of the journey through illness could provide clinicians with the opportunity to tailor the process of diagnosis, treatment, and management to suit the individual's needs (person-centered approach). One way of understanding the journey of the patient is by using the approach of narrative-based medicine. Greenhalgh and Hurwitz (1999) argued, "narratives of illness provide a framework for approaching a patient's problems holistically, and may uncover diagnostic and therapeutic options" (p. 48).

The *patient journey model* can help understand the patient's story (or narrative) in a structured way. It provides an overview of the patient's view on the following: how it feels for an individual to face a hearing loss; how a PHL adapts their life to manage such a condition; positive and negative experiences; and its relationship to quality of life (Manchaiah and Stephens, 2011). The narratives can be used on the one hand to disclose stigmatization and misunderstanding. On the other hand, it can be used to show how a PHL struggles for recognition and refuses to be stigmatized.

Such an approach in studying the patient journey places emphasis on the skills of listening, appreciating, and interpreting the patient's stories, which are key functions during the clinical encounter. It provides very useful anecdotal information at the expense of a structured approach and can be useful in understanding the complex processes underlying acquired hearing loss. In short, it can serve as input in a biopsychosocial understanding of living with hearing loss.

In clinical situations, identifying the experiences that PHLs experience and their psychological state of mind may help the clinician in planning the treatment strategies. Stephens and Kramer (2009) suggest that the patient with hearing loss can be broadly categorized into four groups based on their rehabilitation types, which include: (1) Positively motivated without complicating factors; (2) Positively motivated with complicating factors; (3) Want help, but reject a key component; and (4) Deny any problems. The *patient journey model* can help us to see these patients in the time domain. For example, the patients in category 3 could be in the movement and/or diagnostic phase and the patients in category 4 could be in the pre-awareness phase. For this reason obtaining detailed information about psychosocial aspects of hearing loss additional to the routine objective data obtained through clinical investigations should be encouraged in clinical practice. In addition, studying the patient journey could be very useful in developing care pathways (Layton et al., 1998).

See Chapter 14 for in-depth discussions about implications and practical applications of the *patient journey model*.

ICF and the journey model of person with hearing loss

In the introductory chapter, we mentioned that a biopsychosocial perspective is necessary to fully understand the process of living with hearing loss. The conceptual model of ICF and especially the ICF Core Sets (see Appendix) is important in order to fully include the experiences of the PHL. In the Core Sets, there are a number of categories that highlight different aspects of the journey. It is striking how many of the categories, especially in activity and participation and environment factors are related to the seven phases. Therefore it is important to use these Core Sets when assessing the functioning of PHLs. By using this conceptual model the patient will be given help to articulate relevant experiences and health aspects.

Summary

Living with a chronic loss of functioning (e.g., hearing loss) is a process that can be interpreted and understood as a life-long journey. The term "patient journey" refers to understanding the experiences and the processes that the patient goes through during the course of the disease and the treatment regime. The journey can be analyzed and understood as a number of chronological phases including: (1) Pre-awareness, (2) Awareness, (3) Movement, (4) Diagnostics, (5) Rehabilitation, (6) Self-evaluation, and (7) Resolution. In this chapter, the seven phases were briefly defined and state-of-the-art knowledge regarding the different phases was outlined. However, it is important to note that there may be some cyclic movement back and forth between different phases. It is not always a linear process. In order to illustrate this concept, two cases were presented which illustrate the content of the phases from a PHL horizon. The *patient journey model* can be helpful for clinicians to develop appropriate management strategies during aural rehabilitation.

References

Chia, E., Wang, J., Rochtchina, E., Cumming, R., Newall, P., and Mitchell, P., 2007. Hearing impairment and health-related quality of life: The Blue Mountains hearing study. *Ear and Hearing*, 28(2), pp. 187–195.

Edgett, L., 2002. *Help-seeking for advanced rehabilitation by adults with hearing loss: An ecological model.* Unpublished Doctoral Thesis, University of British Columbia, Vancouver, Canada.

Engelund, G., 2006. *Time for hearing – recognising process for the individual.* Unpublished Doctoral Thesis, University of Copenhagen, Copenhagen, Denmark.

Greenhalgh, T. and Hurwitz, B., 1999. Narrative based medicine: Why study narrative? *British Medical Journal*, 318, pp. 48–50.

Hunt, L. and Arar, N., 2000. An analytical framework for contrasting patient and provider views of the process of chronic disease management. *Medical Anthropology Quarterly*, 15(3), pp. 347–367.

Ida Institute, 2009. A possible patient journey. *Ida Institute* [online]. Available at: http://idainstitute.com/toolbox/ci_resources/self_development/get_started/patient_journey/ [Accessed on 16 March 2016].

Laplante-Lévesque, A., Knudsen, L., Preminger, et al., 2012. Hearing help-seeking and rehabilitation: Perspectives of adults with hearing impairment. *International Journal of Audiology*, 51(2), pp. 93–102.

Laplante-Lévesque, A., Hickson, L., and Worrall, L., 2013. Stages of change in adults with acquired hearing impairment seeking help for the first time: Application of the transtheoretical model in audiologic rehabilitation. *Ear and Hearing*, 34(4), pp. 447–457.

Laplante-Lévesque, A., Brännström, K.J., Ingo, E., Andersson, G., and Lunner, T., 2015. Stages of change in adults who have failed an online hearing screening. *Ear and Hearing*, 36(1), pp. 92–101.

Layton, A., Moss, F., and Morgan, G., 1998. Mapping out the patient's journey: Experiences of developing pathways of care. *Quality in Healthcare*, 7(S2), pp. 30S–36S.

Manchaiah, V., 2012. Health behavior change in hearing healthcare: A discussion paper. *Audiology Research*, 2(4), pp. 12–16.

Manchaiah, V. and Stephens, D., 2011. The patient journey: Living with acquired hearing impairment. *Journal of the Academy of Rehabilitative Audiology*, 44, pp. 29–40.

Manchaiah, V. and Stephens, D., 2012. The patient journey of adults with sudden-onset acquired hearing impairment: A pilot study. *The Journal of Laryngology and Otology*, 126(5), pp. 475–481.

Manchaiah, V., Stephens, D., and Meredith, R., 2011. The patient journey of adults with hearing impairment: The patients' view. *Clinical Otolaryngology*, 36(3), pp. 227–234.

Manchaiah, V., Rönnberg, J., Andersson, G., and Lunner, T., 2015. Stages of change profiles among adults experiencing hearing difficulties who have not taken any action: A cross-sectional study. *PLUS One*, 10(6): e0129107. doi:10.1371/journal.pone.0129107.

Prochaska, J. and DiClemente, C., 1982. Transtheoretical theory: Toward a more integrative model of change. *Psychotherapy: Theory, Research, & Practice*, 19(3), pp. 276–288.

Prochaska, J. O., Johnson, S., and Lee, P., 2009. The transtheoretical model of behavior change. In S. A. Shumaker, J. K. Ockene, and K. A. Riekert (Eds.), *The handbook of health behavior change* (3rd ed., pp. 59–83). New York, NY: Springer.

Stephens, D. and Kramer S., 2009. *Living with hearing difficulties: The process of enablement.* Chichester, West Sussex, UK: John Wiley & Sons, Ltd.

World Health Organization, 2012. *Engage in the process of change: Facts and methods.* WHO Regional Office for Europe, Copenhagen, Denmark: World Health Organization.

4

COMMUNICATION PARTNERS' JOURNEY THROUGH THEIR PARTNER'S HEARING LOSS

Vinaya Manchaiah and Berth Danermark

Introduction

In Chapter 3, the patient journey model of the person with hearing loss (PHL) was presented. In this chapter, the journey model of communication partners (CPs), along with some narratives, is provided.

Defining communication partners

Interpersonal communication is a mutual process, which involves meaningful exchange of information between two or more people. This will be further elaborated in Chapter 11.

Communication is an important part of human society, especially to be able to participate in various social activities. The ability to communicate various emotions, thoughts, and feelings through a verbal medium and general use of language is quite unique to humans. Hence, hearing is a crucial aspect for verbal communication. If you lose your ability to hear, you lose your ability to participate in important activities and relationships, unless you change the mode of communication (e.g., sign language). Therefore, hearing loss is a communication problem that affects everyone in the communication situation, not only the PHL. It can result in various physical, mental, and psychosocial effects on PHLs and their CPs.

The CPs are those with whom the PHL communicates on a regular basis. Often CPs are referred to as significant others, but this term may not properly describe the broad range of partners in communication. Therefore, the term communication partner is used to encompass this wide range of persons, including spouses, siblings, children, friends, relatives, colleagues, and caregivers (Manchaiah et al., 2013).

Third-party disability

According to the World Health Organization (WHO) – International Classification of Functioning, Disability and Health (ICF), third-party disability is defined as the "disability of family members due to the health condition of their significant other" (World Health Organization, 2001). Married CPs of a PHL, although they do not have the health condition themselves, may experience activity limitations and participation restrictions due to their spouse's hearing loss resulting in third-party disability (Scarinci et al., 2009). While spouses of PHLs experience the majority of limitations, the adverse consequences can extend to other CPs (e.g., children, friends, colleagues).

Consequences of hearing loss on communication partners

The experiences of CPs may vary greatly from person to person. However, often CPs may experience various adverse consequences because of their partner's condition (Manchaiah et al., 2012; Scarinci et al., 2008; Stephens et al., 1995). These may include difficulty communicating, changes to relationship, misunderstanding, anger and frustration, social withdrawal and so on (see Table 4.1 for more details). It is noteworthy that, although acquired hearing loss may not be the main cause of the relationship problems between the PHL and the CP, it can add to or exacerbate problems. Nevertheless, although surprising, some positive experiences have also been reported by CPs due to their partner's hearing loss. These may include: personal development (e.g., development of patience and tolerance), improved communication skills, understanding, and awareness of hearing problems and so on.

TABLE 4.1 Effect of hearing disability of person with hearing loss on communication partners (adapted from Danermark, 2014)

Anxiety **Reduced satisfaction** **Reduced quality of social relationships**	• Uncertainty about the future • Difficult to do things together • Loss of close relationships • Reduced socializing with friends
Negative self-image **Tiring**	• Embarrassment • Acting as interpreter • Always answering the telephone • Assistive technology • High volume on the radio and television • Loud speech • Repeating • Speaking clearly, slowly • Speaking one at a time • Using sign language
Positive experiences	• The kindness of others

These positive experiences may be related to the temperament of CPs and their attitudes towards hearing loss and its consequences.

It is commonly reported by CPs that denial of a hearing loss by the PHL often creates conflict among them. While CPs may include other groups of people connected to the PHL (e.g., siblings, children, family, etc.), spouses are the most common CP. When spouses are the CP, there is a risk for crisis due to the effects of hearing loss. This frustration and anxiety may lead to behavior and coping strategies that are often maladaptive. Such crisis can be defined as an emotionally significant event that is frequently the turning point, for better or worse, for a given situation. Hence, PHLs who are in denial may be in a constant state of crisis with their spouse and family. Recognizing this crisis and making a commitment to address problems may result in more harmonious relationships. Moreover, CPs may also be in need of help and rehabilitation to cope with their third-party disability (Preminger and Meeks, 2010).

Role of communication partners in aural rehabilitation

Only a small number of PHLs are self-motivated to seek help for their hearing loss. However, many end up in audiology clinics due to pressure from CPs persuading them to seek help (Duijvestijn et al., 2003). It is therefore reasonable to assume that the behavior of the CP may play an important role in the decision of the PHL to seek a consultation and accept intervention. In addition, it is understood that if patient expectations are not met with hearing aids, they become disappointed and frustrated (Donaldson et al., 2004). CPs provide support and encouragement to PHLs by acting as an interpreter and providing emotional assistance. This helps to bridge the gap between the partner's expectations and hearing aid performance.

CPs may undergo various experiences through their partner's hearing loss and this may often influence the help-seeking behaviors of the PHL. However, if the CP does not understand the impact of hearing loss on the PHL's life, it is very unlikely that they will be able to support them. Hence, it is very important to involve CPs during the audiological enablement and rehabilitation process, which may result in mutual advantages for both the PHL and their CPs (Manchaiah et al., 2012).

Stephens and Kramer (2009) suggest that aural rehabilitation is an active process (i.e., enablement). The audiological enablement should focus on enhancing the activities and participation of individuals with hearing loss, improving their quality of life, and minimizing the effects on CPs. Their recommended approach includes four main stages: (1) evaluation, (2) integration and decision making, (3) short-term remediation, and (4) ongoing remediation. To adopt such an approach, it is essential to gain deeper understanding of the consequences of hearing loss on the lives of PHLs and CPs, the positive and negative experiences reported, and the journey they experience during the course of their condition. Stephens and Kramer (2009) also suggest that the key components of the non-instrumental intervention strategy should involve goal setting, involvement of CPs, and hearing tactics. This model can provide some insights to involvement of CPs in the aural rehabilitation process.

Communication partners' journey

The Ida Institute in Denmark, with collaborative effort from hearing healthcare professionals around the world, developed the possible CP journey model. However, this model was based only on professional perspectives and included six main phases: (1) contemplation, (2) awareness, (3) persuasion, (4) validation, (5) rehabilitation, and (6) maintenance. It was suggested that this model recognizes the emotional reactions and practical activities the CPs experience during the onset of their partner's hearing loss, successful management, and learning to live with the condition.

Studies from medical anthropologists (Hunt and Arar, 2000) and from studies of the patient journey of PHLs have shown differences in professional and patient perspectives (Manchaiah et al., 2011). This may indicate that the professional and CP perception of the CP journey could also be different. Hence, CPs' views were considered to further develop the CP journey model (Manchaiah et al., 2013). Figure 4.1 shows the typical journey model of CPs, which has seven main phases: (1) contemplation, (2) awareness, (3) persuasion, (4) validation, (5) rehabilitation, (6) adaptation, and (7) resolution. These phases correspond quite well with stages of change in the transtheoretical model of change (TTM), which demonstrates an individual's readiness to act on new health behavior (Prochaska and Velicer, 1997), and also with the journey of PHL (Manchaiah et al., 2011). Moreover, a new phase, *adaptation*, was identified from the CPs' view, which was not identified by hearing healthcare professionals as reported by the Ida Institute (2010) possible partner journey.

In this chapter, the phases of the CP journey are presented in a temporal order. In research, there was some temporal order to CP narratives regarding the journey, but not all the CPs reported them in order (Manchaiah et al., 2013). For example, CPs may go back and forth in phases while talking about their journey. This may be due to their inability to remember the fine details and thoroughly articulate the experiences that may have influenced this. There may be some overlap in phases and the time spent in each phase may vary markedly from person to person (i.e., several days to several years). In addition, it is almost impossible to precisely identify which phase the CPs may be in at one point in time. Hence, seeing the journey as a continuum and as a process is necessary. Moreover, some experiences can be seen in multiple phases. For example, role sharing and relationship dynamics were reported both in initial and later phases

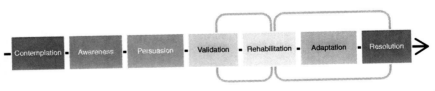

FIGURE 4.1 Main phases of communication partners' journey through their partner's hearing loss (taken from Manchaiah et al., 2013 with permission from Hindawi Publishing Corporation)

of the journey. CPs talked more about contemplation, awareness, adaptation, and resolution phases compared to other phases (i.e., persuasion, validation, and rehabilitation).

The following details the seven phases of the CP journey and provides some narrative accounts to better illustrate them (Manchaiah et al., 2013). It is important to note that the CP journey runs in parallel with the journey of PHLs. See Chapter 1 to explore the differences and similarities in the journey of PHLs and CPs.

Contemplation

In the contemplation phase (e.g., "what is going on?"), CPs may start noticing the PHL's communication difficulties and reduced social interactions. This may sometimes result in feeling embarrassed, angry, and frustrated. Initially the CPs might attribute some of the problems noticed to possible cognitive impairments, attention, or concentration issues. Moreover, the CPs may also start making some accommodations for the PHL's hearing difficulties.

The following statement made by the CP of a PHL shows how, in the initial phase of the PHL's hearing loss, the CP may think that the communication difficulties noticed were due to attention and concentration rather than to poor hearing. This highlights the fact that identification of hearing loss is not straightforward.

> Initially I thought a lot of it was due to his attention! I could say something to him and if it was not of his interest, I could see that he has not heard it, or he will repeat what I said five minutes later, and I would say, I just told you that! Even though I had experience with deafness due to others in the family, I could not realize he had a problem straightaway.

Awareness

In the awareness phase, CPs become aware that the PHL has genuine hearing difficulties. This may be by noticing clear changes in the PHL's communication behavior, the PHL's dependency on other senses, noticing that the PHL was not hearing alerting signals (e.g., smoke alarm, telephone ringing, etc.), and, more importantly, by noticing changes in the family dynamics. They may start nagging the PHL, indirectly persuading the PHL to seek help, providing support and encouragement, and may start acting as an interpreter for the PHL. However, this new role of acting as an interpreter may become overwhelming.

This description below shows how a CP confirmed their speculation about the PHL's hearing loss, with elements of contemplation and awareness phases. It also highlights how awareness may change family dynamics.

> I can remember a few things, which can put the picture together ... the first thing I noticed was that he was shouting on the telephone. I could be in there

with the doors shut and could hear him. I say to him, do you realize that you were shouting on the telephone? I don't think I was ... You can't say anything to that one ... and the other thing is shouting at public places, for example, shouting in the restaurant ... after it was confirmed to me with these observations, I told my children what I noticed, and they agreed, especially the elder daughter, and she started making some adjustments ...

The following statement made by a CP highlights the change in their communication roles, a change in family dynamics, and the dependency of the PHL on the CP for everyday activities in relation to communication.

After I started noticing his difficulties ... I almost started acting like his secretary ... it could be very tiring sometimes ... especially later in the day ...!

Persuasion

After CPs become aware of the PHL's hearing loss they often start making attempts to make the PHL aware of their communication problems. In addition, they may also start searching for information related to hearing loss and start persuading them to seek help. In the initial stages, this could be indirect. However, there could be some triggering factors for the CPs, which makes them start directly persuading the PHL to seek help.

The following quote confirms that the CPs could act as drivers (or facilitators) to the PHL seeking help. The CP's expression makes it clear that this task is not always straightforward. They may start with indirect persuasion and move to persuasion that is more direct as time progresses.

I have to be very diplomatic you know. [chuckle] I got a bit of adverse reaction on one occasion. He said to me, speak up you are mumbling, and I said to him, you are not hearing me properly and asked him to get his hearing checked ... [chuckle] He said to me, you get your hearing checked; you don't hear something that I say to you ... Once he said that, I have to back off for a while obviously ... work with it for a while and then change my approach ... I think I nagged him to such an extent that he went to get a hearing test ... he was not hearing the telephone, once he did not hear the alarm and ... once it got to that stage, I have to tell him!

Validation

This phase was not widely discussed by the CPs. However, in this phase CPs mainly confirm whether the PHL has hearing loss. The results of hearing assessment of the PHLs may or may not surprise the CPs. Even though most CPs are not very keen about the hearing assessment, some accompany the PHL and make an attempt to understand the hearing test results and what they may indicate. However, almost all make commitments to support the PHLs.

In this statement, the CP talks about the PHL's reaction to the hearing test and acceptance of hearing loss. However, this also indirectly implies that the CP confirmed that their assessment was correct. There are also elements of later stages being mentioned, for example, the rehabilitation phase (i.e., starting to wear hearing aids).

> After the hearing test, the realization made him do something about it … after he consulted he started wearing hearing aids, getting them fixed regularly, adjusts them, and it has made a great difference to us.

Rehabilitation

In this phase, most CPs were relieved that the PHLs were seeking help. However, they start realizing that they also have an important role to play in the rehabilitation process, mainly in supporting the PHL (e.g., in using hearing aids). They may realize that hearing instruments will not solve all the problems, which makes them feel sympathy for the PHL's difficulties.

The following description highlights that, soon after the PHL is fitted with hearing aids, they will discover that hearing aids do not solve all communication difficulties. In addition, the coping strategies used and the way in which the CP would support the PHL are evident.

> He wears hearing aids, but I still have to shout and I say things six times … oh … I have to say six times very often! You hear what I said then? … He will say no … oh … right … I will start again then. So, it's again my temperament … I don't get cross over him. I would say … oh … for goodness sake … you listening now? [chuckle] … watch my lips … [chuckle] …

The following statement made by a CP is an example of what may happen at a dinner table during a big family dinner. This may suggest that they feel sorry for the PHL, as they feel helpless on some occasions.

> I feel a bit guilty sometimes … Everyone having a conversation … having a laugh and everything … I feel guilty sometime if he can't join in sometime, and if he is sitting in the corner … and everyone don't realize that.

Adaptation

Adaptation was a new phase identified from CP reports when compared to the Ida Institute professionals' perspectives of the communication partners' journey (Ida Institute, 2010). This phase was noticed soon after the hearing assessment and rehabilitation session, when CPs started exploring new ways to communicate with the PHL, adapting to regular role sharing, and reflecting on positive and negative consequences of the hearing impairment and the audiological management. Many elderly CPs also report beginning to notice hearing problems themselves and comparing their own problems to those of the PHL.

The spouse of a PHL made the following statement in relation to how they started exploring new ways of communication after he was confirmed as having hearing loss.

> I do repeat things for him, yes, he said such and such … sometime he will ask me what did he say, when he misses a bit … the other day I repeated three times and eventually I say, I spell it out … because if they don't get it after three times … then we just spell it out.

The following quote was made while a CP was talking about how he adapted to dealing with the PHL, demonstrating that the CP was able to identify some positive aspects of hearing loss.

> It's not like he is missing a lot, because we talk after the meeting, what has been said, and it's not like he is missing anything. In fact, there is another person in the office who just can't be bothered, who goes to meeting and … dreams. Whereas he [name of PHL] is different, he concentrates on what is being said and pays attention. Maybe it's been a benefit to him in that respect, because, he is hard of hearing so he has got to concentrate on hearing it.

Resolution

This has been identified as a more a stable phase that most CPs reported during the course of interviews. In this phase, CPs note continued difficulties experienced by the PHL in social situations and began to realize that the crisis may not necessarily be hearing related. They also gradually begin to notice the increasing difficulties of the PHL, possibly due to worsening of their hearing loss. Some CPs with positive temperaments report satisfactory outcomes. However, others report frustration and disappointing outcomes. Changes in family relationships seemed like a dynamic process, which was noticed even in this phase. Moreover, in this phase most CPs were more stable and hearing loss had just become a way of life compared to the earlier phase (i.e., adaptation) in which they were exploring new ways of communication to improve the situation.

The following statement illustrates how the CP has started using a certain way of communicating rather than exploring new ways of communication.

> We have a way of talking to him now. We have a certain way. We sometime do it with normal hearing people when I talk to them, and they say why are you speaking to me like this? I am so used to being around dad. It does change our lives.

A daughter of a PHL made this statement indicating how her life had changed and the crisis was not only hearing related.

> It's our responsibility now ... because we can't expect him to do everyday things now. He will pick up the phone and ring me. Nine out of ten times, he does not understand what we say. Few times now, since my mother has died and he lives on his own, if we don't get a response from him on the telephone we have to go there to check if he's alright.

Clinical implications of the communication partners' journey

The CP journey model helps to see the "bigger picture" about experiences of CPs and how they change over time, which is most important in managing chronic conditions (e.g., hearing loss). Since this model is organized chronologically, a format often used in storytelling, it is relatively easy for both professionals and non-professionals to understand and remember. The narrative (i.e., storytelling/listening) approach is a simple and useful way to gather data from CPs. We suggest that this model could be helpful for clinicians to identify which phase (e.g., contemplation, awareness, persuasion) the CPs might be in during clinical encounters by taking an in-depth case history. This model should assist clinicians in helping patients think about their journey. Clinicians can begin case history discussions by asking CPs to describe their stories. Understanding how the experiences of CPs change over time and in what phases they are presently in could be important for clinicians during counseling in order to tailor the information provided to meet the individual CP's needs.

The identification of a new phase (i.e., adaptation) is important in terms of clinical practice that may highlight the need for review appointments soon after the initial assessment and rehabilitation session. These review sessions should be focused on assessing and modifying expectations, providing psychosocial support, and teaching communication tactics to CPs (Manchaiah et al., 2013). Moreover, it is important for hearing healthcare professionals to understand the journey of both the PHLs and their CPs in order to facilitate their partnership during audiological enablement/rehabilitation. For this reason, the CP journey model should be used in training hearing healthcare professionals.

ICF and the journey model of communication partners

From a dialogue perspective of communication, the crucial aspect is the creation of meaning within interaction (for further discussion, see Chapter 11). The implication is that the most significant aspect of living with hearing loss and the journey cannot be understood without considering the CP. Interacting with others is a significant part in all of the phases. This becomes obvious when looking at which categories are included in the Core Sets, where categories such as conversation, family relationships, intimate relationships, immediate and extended family, basic and complex interpersonal interactions are included (see Appendix). In employment, community life and political life as well as interacting with health services, it is not possible to understand the communication aspect without including the CP.

Summary

In this chapter, we have brought the CP to the forefront. Interpersonal communication is a mutual process and hence the process of living with hearing loss cannot be understood without including the CP. We have defined CPs as those with whom the PHL communicates on a regular basis. These can be family members, friends, work peers, or professionals in health services. It must be acknowledged that a hearing loss has consequences for the CP, especially the "significant others." A number of negative consequences (e.g., loss of close relationships, difficulty of doing things together, embarrassment) have been listed, but some positive ones such as the kindness of others were also included. Research has shown that it is very important to involve CPs during the audiological enablement and rehabilitation process. It is not only the PHL that experiences a journey, but also the CP. Seven main phases were discussed, including: (1) contemplation, (2) awareness, (3) persuasion, (4) validation, (5) rehabilitation, (6) adaptation, and (7) resolution. The CP journey model can be useful in professional education and patient counseling.

References

Danermark, B., 2014. *(Re)capturing the conversation: A book about hearing loss and communication.* New Delhi, Delhi: Kanishka Publishers and Distributors.

Donaldson, N., Worrall, L., and Hickson, L., 2004. Older people with hearing impairment: A literature review of the spouse's perspective. *Australia and New Zealand Journal of Audiology*, 26(1), pp. 30–39.

Duijvestijn, J., Anteunis, L., Hoek C., et al., 2003. Help-seeking behaviour of hearing-impaired persons aged 55 years: Effect of complaints, significant others, and hearing aid image. *Acta Oto-laryngologica*, 123(7), pp. 846–850.

Hunt, L. and Arar, N., 2000. An analytical framework for contrasting patient and provider views of the process of chronic disease management. *Medical Anthropology Quarterly*, 15(3), pp. 347–367.

Ida Institute, 2009. A possible patient journey. *Ida Institute* [online]. Available at: http://idainstitute.com/toolbox/ci_resources/self_development/get_started/patient_journey/ [Accessed on 16 March 2016].

Ida Institute, 2010. A possible partner journey. *Ida Institute* [online]. Available at: http://idainstitute.com/toolbox/communication_partners/get_started/partner_journey/ [Accessed on 16 August 2016].

Manchaiah, V., Stephens, D., and Meredith, R., 2011. The patient journey of adults with hearing impairment: The patients' view. *Clinical Otolaryngology*, 36(3), pp. 227–234.

Manchaiah, V., Stephens, D., Zhao, F., et al., 2012. The role of communication partners in the audiological enablement/rehabilitation of a person with hearing impairment: A discussion paper. *Audiological Medicine*, 10(6), pp. 21–30.

Manchaiah, V. Stephens, D., and Lunner, T., 2013. Communication partners' journey through their partner's hearing impairment. *International Journal of Otolaryngology*, pp. 1–11.

Preminger, J. and Meeks, S., 2010. Evaluation of an audiological rehabilitation program for spouses of people with hearing loss. *Journal of the American Academy of Audiology*, 21(5), pp. 315–328.

Prochaska, J. and Velicer, W., 1997. The transtheoretical model of health behaviour change. *American Journal of Health Promotion*, 12(1), pp. 38–48.

Scarinci, N., Worrall, L., and Hickson, L., 2008. The effect of hearing impairment in older people on the spouse. *International Journal of Audiology*, 47(3), pp. 141–151.

Scarinci, N., Worrall, L., and Hickson, L., 2009. The ICF and third-party disability: Its application to spouses of older people with hearing impairment. *Disability Rehabilitation*, 31(25), pp. 2088–2100.

Stephens, D. and Kramer S., 2009. *Living with hearing difficulties: The process of enablement.* Chichester, West Sussex, UK: John Wiley & Sons, Ltd.

Stephens, D., France, L., and Lormore, K., 1995. Effects of impairment on the patient's family and friends. *Acta Oto-laryngologica*, 115(2), pp. 165–167.

World Health Organization, 2001. *International Classification of Functioning, Disability and Health (ICF)*. Geneva, Switzerland: World Health Organization.

5

PRE-AWARENESS

Failing to notice or realize hearing loss

Samuel Trychin

Introduction

In previous chapters, the ideas of *process of change*, *patient journey*, and *process evaluation* were presented. From this chapter on, a detailed understanding of the phases of the journey, which includes both the actors, the person with hearing loss (PHL) and communication partners (CPs), and the process will be discussed. This chapter presents the first phase, *pre-awareness*. It is important to note that not much literature exists on this pre-clinical phase, as most of the literature is on the clinical population.

Our sense of hearing

Staying in tune with events in the environment is essential for survival on Planet Earth. We must be aware of things that are threatening or dangerous in order to avoid or escape them. Conversely, we must be aware of things that are beneficial in order to approach and acquire them. Fortunately, we are born with mechanisms that allow us to detect these events either consciously or subconsciously and then respond appropriately to them.

For events nearby, we have sensory systems that provide information about their presence. Taste, smell, and touch receptors all function to provide information about things we need to avoid or acquire that are nearby. Vision and hearing senses provide information about events both nearby and at a distance that we need to avoid or approach.

Hearing can be considered our most important distance sense to keep us informed about events happening in our environment. Hearing and vision alert us to events occurring in front and to the sides of us. Unlike vision, however, hearing alerts us to events occurring behind us, around corners, and to those hidden behind objects. Additionally, hearing continues to function while we are asleep while vision is greatly diminished when our eyes are closed (Horowitz, 2012).

When there is a malfunction in any of the sensory systems, we are deprived of the information provided by that system. For example, when a person does not have normal sense of touch, a highly controlled environment is often necessary to help keep the person out of danger, healthy, and alive. Loss of ability to hear environmental sounds, including speech, deprives the individual of important information necessary for both physical and psychological health.

Most of the "moment-to-moment" information processed by our nervous system and brain is not occurring at the conscious level, but at much lower, subconscious levels. For example, unless we focus attention on the ticking of a clock, we are often not aware of its sound. It is to our survival benefit that we are largely unconscious of all the stimulation that is occurring constantly around and within us. Attending consciously to the repetitive sounds of our breathing and all environmental noises occurring around us would be exhausting and would make it difficult to focus on much more important issues.

However, having these internal and external environmental sounds registering at subconscious levels is necessary for normal functioning and, perhaps, survival. When there is a *change* in these stimuli, it attracts our attention, indicating that we may need to focus on the cause of the change and do something. For example, when the usual sounds of the car engine change, it is wise to check for the cause. When the sound of the baby's breathing pattern is altered, it is time to check on him/her.

It can be more obvious when having difficulty hearing sounds that are processed at a more conscious level (e.g., your boss's voice during an important meeting), as this might create life difficulties. While driving, an inability to determine the location of the blaring of a fire engine's siren might produce apprehension. Concerns that you might not hear the sound of the alarm clock or the telephone in your hotel room while away at a conference might cause some anxiety.

It may be much less obvious when missing sounds that are processed at the subconscious level; but this also creates negative emotional and physical effects. It is likely that the sensory void created by less than normal hearing, at even milder levels of deficit, can result in chronic apprehension or anxiety. This in turn, even at lower levels, can have a negative effect on energy, mood, and health. Connecting these negative experiences to hearing problems is uncommon, and thus the hearing loss often goes unrecognized. In fact, most people fail to notice or take steps to manage and cope with their hearing loss. Reasons for this have been identified (Trychin, 1990), including that the PHL:

- does not:
  - realize they have problems hearing;
  - want to admit to having problems hearing;
  - recognize the relationship between their hearing loss and their emotional, social, and physical problems/status;
  - know where to turn to get help;
  - have access to hearing care providers;
  - have the money to pay for hearing services/equipment;
- has other, more pressing problems in their lives to deal with.

In this chapter, the focus is on that group of people who have hearing loss but are unaware of its presence – those who are at a *preconscious* level (i.e., pre-awareness phase). For many people, hearing loss begins at low levels and increases gradually in small increments over time. Such people habituate to each new level of hearing loss until it becomes noticeable to them or to others who bring it to their attention. Some others remaining unaware of their hearing loss may have psychological, emotional, or social reasons for their unwillingness to recognize that the hearing loss is present. The mechanism for this is sometimes referred to as *denial*, but care should be taken when resorting to denial as the only explanation, as it is an overused and often inaccurate explanation. For discussion about awareness, acknowledgment, and acceptance of hearing loss, see Chapter 6.

Alcock (2015) lists several reasons other than denial why people who have hearing loss may fail to realize its presence. First, when a sound is below the hearing threshold, it simply does not exist for the PHL who will not be aware of or "miss" its presence. Second, all people have experienced dealing with poor auditory signals (e.g., speaker's too low or too fast speech, noisy background or echo sounds, signal source too far away), and so they manage the difficulty hearing as they always have when the listening situation is less than ideal. Third, people with high frequency hearing loss often hear low frequency sounds well and take that as evidence that their hearing is normal. Fourth, people use information from other sources, like vision or cognition (e.g., using a speaker's facial expression and body language; usual language patterns), to fill in gaps in the auditory signal.

Alcock (2015) also lists several reasons why so many people with hearing loss fail to take action to increase their ability to hear. First, is the lack of evidence of the loss of their ability to hear normally. Most people do not have a baseline record of their previous hearing level to compare with their current level of hearing. Second, other people who do notice that the person is not hearing very well may compensate for it by speaking louder and/or slowing their rate of speech. Third, some people look for evidence that indicates their hearing is normal (e.g., hearing quite well in a quiet area while speaking with only one other person).

Hearing loss is a communication disorder and, as such, it affects all people involved in a communicative exchange, both the PHL and their CPs. When a CP is unaware that hearing loss is present, changes, even subtle changes, in their partner with hearing loss can be attributed to other things (e.g., inattention, dementia, or personality problems). The following four case examples illustrate how hearing loss undetected or denied can negatively affect the PHL and CPs.

Examples illustrating the effects of unnoticed hearing loss

Scenario one

This scenario illustrates the problems due to lack of awareness/failure to notice hearing loss.

George is unaware of the subtle increments in his inability to hear normally. This scenario discusses the possible physical, emotional, cognitive, and social effects.

At home

Effects on self: George feels less energy than he had earlier in his life, but attributes his tiredness to becoming older and having more responsibilities at home and work. He also feels that he is not as sharp at work as he had been earlier in his life, but thinks he just needs to get more sleep at night. George hasn't attended the weekly card game with his buddies for the past several months because he believes he just isn't getting the same pleasure from being with them that he once did, and he doesn't want to leave his wife alone to care for the kids, chores, etc. George feels somewhat down these days, but also attributes this to his increasing lack of energy and need for more sleep.

Effects on spouse: George's wife, Melissa, is increasingly concerned about his apparent lack of interest in her and the children. He often fails to respond to her questions or comments and does not regularly watch TV with the family as he once did. In the past, Melissa and George often shared funny or interesting experiences each had during the day and did so while working in different rooms, e.g., she in her office and he in the kitchen. That sharing of experiences has largely stopped. Melissa is becoming increasingly concerned that George might be having an affair with someone else and finds herself becoming increasingly depressed and irritable (Trychin, 2014a).

Effects on children: The kids, ages two and four, like to play active games, talking and yelling while running around the house. It is hard to get them to sit still for very long while talking with them. Their voices are high pitched, sometimes shrill, and can be difficult to understand. It is particularly difficult when their faces are turned away. Both children feel let down when Dad does not stop what he is doing to play with them or tell stories and answer their questions. He has just been too busy doing other things and has not been around them as much as before. They miss him.

At work

George's supervisor, Roger, is increasingly concerned about George's attitude, motivation, and ability to continue working at the level required for his position in the company. Roger has noticed that George does not seem to be paying sufficient attention during the weekly business meetings. In addition, some of George's coworkers have complained that he is not keeping up with the work he needs to do in order for them to do their own jobs. Some of his coworkers feel that George is not always listening to what they ask him to do, especially when down in the machine shop.

Scenario two

This scenario illustrates problems due to unwillingness to admit to hearing loss.

In this case, Dale, as a child, witnessed some verbal abuse and neglect experienced by an elderly aunt who had an obvious hearing loss. He also saw a primary school classmate being teased and bullied because of wearing hearing aids in school. These early experiences have reinforced Dale's stereotypic view that people who have hearing loss are weaker, more infirm, and more dependent than people who have more or less normal hearing ability. Self-stereotyping has resulted in Dale knowing he has difficulty hearing in some situations but avoiding taking steps to constructively deal with the hearing loss. This scenario discusses the possible physical, emotional, cognitive, and social effects on Dale. This scenario has some overlap in pre-awareness and awareness phases of the journey. For further discussion about awareness and acceptance of hearing loss, see Chapter 6.

At home

Effects on self: Dale is unmarried and lives alone in a condominium. He has had several, brief relationships with women that ended in large part due to his emotional difficulties. He has a history of periodic high anxiety often followed by a depression caused by the exhausting effects on his body of the physical underpinnings of the anxiety.

Dale resorts to *bluffing*, pretending to understand, as his primary coping strategy when he is aware that he does not understand what someone is saying to him. He nods his head, smiles, and says things such as, "uh huh," "right," or "got it." This strategy results in a double dose of anxiety. The first results from failing to understand what the person is saying and the possible negative consequences of that. The second source of his anxiety is fear of being found out – that others will know that he has hearing loss and devalue him (Gagné et al., 2009).

The efforts required of Dale to conceal the fact of his hearing loss and the attendant emotional reactions have taken a toll on his physical health and result in chronic fatigue, which, itself, makes him vulnerable to the emotional ups and downs and to difficulty focusing attention on what others are saying to him.

At work

Dale's job mostly entails working alone on his computer, but also requires random interactions with coworkers and supervisors during the workday. He is able to avoid the social gatherings around the coffee area at break times by continuing to work during that time. His coworkers think he is not very friendly and mostly leave him alone during the break periods. Dale experiences some anxiety during the conversations with coworkers/supervisors during the day due to concern that if his hearing difficulties are discovered, he might lose his job.

Scenario three

This scenario illustrates the problems due to lack of information about hearing loss, resulting in misdiagnosis and failure to remediate the true source of the problems.

Grandma Gresham has gradual onset, bilateral hearing loss, which has not been diagnosed. Mrs. Gresham had been living alone for several years following her husband's death. She moved into a nursing home about a year ago and has recently become increasingly socially isolated and depressed. The staff and Mrs. Gresham's family members are concerned about her deteriorating physical and psychological condition. This scenario discusses the possible physical, emotional, cognitive, and social effects:

On grandma Gresham: When she first arrived at the nursing home, Mrs. Gresham, age 89, enjoyed the interactions she had with other residents and the staff. It was a welcome and stimulating experience after having been living alone much of the time. However, her undiagnosed hearing loss was increasing to the point that she was having difficulty understanding what others were saying. Negative reactions to her communication difficulties from some other residents resulted in Mrs. Gresham feeling unwelcome. That and the added experience of several painfully embarrassing situations in which she had misunderstood what was said resulted in feelings of shame.

Social pain often results when a person feels left out, rejected, or in some other way separated from someone or a group of people who are of importance to that person. Social pain is real and has a neural basis in the brain that is part of the same neural network that underlies physical pain (McDonald and Jensen-Campbell, 2011).

In order to reduce the painful feelings associated with embarrassment and shame, Mrs. Gresham purposefully isolated herself from the other residents and, as much as possible, from the staff. That strategy helped Mrs. Gresham avoid embarrassing situations, but produced loneliness and resultant depression. Loneliness results in increased physical health problems and, when unchecked, early mortality (Cacioppo, 2003). For further discussion on the secondary effects (i.e., loneliness and depression) of long-term hearing loss, see Chapter 12.

On staff who work with her: The nursing home staff did not have adequate education/training about hearing loss and its effects and, therefore, have been trying to explain Mrs. Gresham's more recent decline as being due to age-related dementia. Medical staff concurred that the depression and increasing social withdrawal were most likely due to some form of a brain-deterioration caused dementia, which is largely untreatable. The treatment prescribed was focused on keeping Mrs. Gresham nourished and ensuring proper hygiene and rest.

On family members: The only family that remained within a comfortable driving distance to the nursing home was a grandson and his wife and two children. When Mrs. Gresham first moved into the nursing home, they had visited her for an hour or two about once every week. Since she had become less communicative and diagnosed with dementia, they have only stopped by twice for brief 15-minute visits.

Scenario four

This scenario illustrates the problems due to lack of information/understanding about a person's hearing loss by others in that person's social environment resulting in misattribution of that person's behavior and social rejection.

A minister's wife, Kate, has profound unilateral hearing loss (UHL) in her right ear and is unable to hear sounds originating from that side. A problem has appeared for the minister and his wife because some members of the church are unhappy with them and want the minister to resign and go somewhere else to preach. Many other members support the minister and his wife and want them to stay. This split in the congregation has produced significant tension and resulted in some members leaving the church altogether.

This problem surfaced during a weeklong workshop the author conducted for people who have hearing loss and their CPs at Ghost Ranch in Abiquiu, New Mexico. Kate was attending the workshop and toward the end of the week exclaimed, "I think I see the cause of the problem." It turns out that she was right and the problem was ultimately resolved leaving the congregation united and happier. The following is what had been happening.

When coming to church, most people sit in the same pew where they have been sitting for many years. Sometimes, families sit in the same location for several generations. People enter the front door of the church and turn right or left, depending on the location of where they sit. The minister and his Kate stand at the center of the entrance area of the church to greet people as they enter. If they go to the right side of the church, they are on the side of Kate's *good* ear, and she hears them and responds to what they say. If they go to the left side, they are on the side of her *bad* ear, and Kate fails to hear them and does not respond to their greeting. The result is that some members believe that the minister and his wife have favorites among the congregation and want them to leave because of that.

At that point in the workshop, Kate told us that she had always tried to hide the fact of her hearing condition. She had feared that it might be seen as something negative, resulting in lowering evaluations of her and her husband's performance as church leaders. A month or two after the workshop ended, the author received a letter from Kate stating that she had written a full-page article in the church bulletin, explaining about her hearing condition and the probable consequences resulting from not informing the congregation about it previously. That article had the effect of resolving the problem and of having many people asking what they might do to be helpful to Kate.

Discussion

These real-life examples (with names changed for privacy) illustrate the difficulties that people experience when someone has less than normal hearing and there is a lack of awareness of its presence. Difficulties are experienced by the PHL, the CPs, or both.

Difficulties can occur in the PHL's *behavior* (e.g., failure to do what has been requested at work or prescribed by a health care provider). Difficulties occur at the *cognitive* level when someone misunderstands what has been said and believes what was heard is correct. Difficulties occur at the *physical* level when, for example, problems caused by hearing loss create a chronic level of tension that results in insufficient sleep. Difficulties occur at the *emotional* level when the person becomes depressed due to losing status at work because of reduced ability to hear. Difficulties occur at the *social* level when a person perceives a loss of an important relationship resulting in social pain and loneliness due to hearing loss. These examples can be expanded to include a host of other behavioral, cognitive, physical, social, and emotional difficulties. Hence, there is a great need to adopt a biopsychosocial approach in understanding and addressing consequences of hearing loss (see Chapter 2).

Difficulties are also experienced by CPs who are unaware that the person has hearing problems and are trying to make sense of what they are experiencing. *Behaviorally*, they may act as though the person is slow-witted, cognitively damaged, or developmentally delayed. *Cognitively*, they may have thoughts that the person is not interested in what they are saying. *Physically*, they may experience increased tension when trying to get the person to understand something important. *Emotionally*, they may experience irritation/anger when the person fails to comply with a request. *Socially*, they may try to avoid and/or escape from any interactions with the person who has hearing loss.

Since at this preconscious level (i.e., pre-awareness phase), there is little or no awareness of the presence of hearing loss, information and support are necessary in helping the PHL come to terms with awareness and acceptance. Information can include signs and symptoms of hearing loss and the fact that it is a communication disorder affecting both speakers and listeners. Information can include problems reported by other people who have hearing loss and by their CP.

At a later point, when there is acceptance of the fact of the hearing loss, communication strategies can be discussed. Information may include the causes of communication breakdowns – speaker, listener, and environmental causes, and communication behavior guidelines for speakers and guidelines for listeners that, when followed, reduce communication hassles. Providing information about and practice in using assistive alerting and listening technology is also helpful at this later stage of awareness.

As indicated in these scenarios, hearing loss is a communication disorder affecting everyone in the communicative situation. The list of problems reported by CPs is as equally lengthy as the list of problems reported by PHLs (Trychin, 2014b). Depending on the importance of the communication situation and the relationship between the person speaking and the person listening, communication difficulties can produce emotional reactivity.

There is evidence that high emotional arousal "shuts down" the functioning of the language centers in the brain, making it difficult to think clearly (McCraty, 2001). The result is that it becomes increasingly difficult to find a solution to the problem or issue that caused the arousal. In the case of problems related to hearing loss, it is essential that the people involved determine the cause of the communication breakdown to suggest and then implement a solution. Negative emotional reactions interfere with making that determination.

However, many people who have hearing loss and their CPs are not aware of the various causes of communication breakdowns, including speaker, listener, and environmental causes (Trychin, 2013). Lacking this information, they are unable to prevent or reduce many of the communication difficulties they experience. On the other hand, there are people who are able to pinpoint the cause(s) of a communication problem, but fail to ask the person speaking to alter some aspect of their communication (e.g., "Can you please speak a little louder when you are talking?").

For some, they may know how but fail to make a request, because they feel it is *impolite* to do so. For example, Sarah reported being quite upset at a dinner party she attended with a group of friends. She said that her hearing loss prevented her from understanding what was being said around the dinner table, so she was unable to participate in the conversation. Sarah said a large flower arrangement directly in front of her prevented her from seeing the faces of the other women across the table and that music was playing at a loud volume, interfering with her ability to understand what the others were saying. When asked why Sarah hadn't requested that the flower arrangement be moved and ask that the stereo volume be turned down, she replied, "Oh, I couldn't do that; it wouldn't be polite!" When asked if sitting there pretending to understand and not participating was more polite, Sarah responded that *she had not thought of it that way.* Thinking more about the situation, Sarah agreed that it really would be more polite to ask for the necessary accommodations and be able to show interest and participate in the conversation.

People who have hearing loss and their frequent CPs can be greatly helped by understanding the different effects that hearing loss can have on communication. In some circumstances (e.g., one-on-one, quiet background, sitting close together), the person who has hearing difficulties can understand perfectly what the other person is saying. In other circumstances (e.g., background noise, poor lighting, or person speaking mumbles), he or she may have much greater difficulty.

When CPs do not know the various causes of communication breakdowns, they may be confused when the PHL understands easily sometimes, but not at all at other times. That often results in such statements as: "You can understand me when you want to" or "You have selective hearing." Neither of these comments serves to nourish relationships.

Both speakers and listeners need to know the difference between *not understanding* and *misunderstanding*. If you say something to me and I am aware that I did not understand what you said, I can easily correct the situation. If I know the reason I did not understand (e.g., you talked too softly or rapidly, I was not paying enough attention, or there was too much background noise), then I can suggest a solution to better understand what you are saying.

If, however, I thought I understood what you said, but actually did not understand correctly, I will have *misunderstood*. Misunderstandings cause many problems both for the person speaking who assumes that the message was understood and for the listener who believes he or she really did understand. For example, you hand your boss a needed contract two days late because you misunderstood the deadline; or a student fails an exam because he or she misunderstood which chapters were to be tested. The best way to prevent misunderstandings is to repeat back, or in some way examine the key elements of what someone has said (e.g., names, dates, numbers, etc.).

Living more easily and successfully with hearing loss requires that both the PHL and their CPs have information necessary for preventing or reducing communication hassles. Living well with hearing loss also requires opportunities to practice new and different ways of communicating that they are learning, along with opportunities to receive feedback about the effectiveness of their efforts. Neither of these requirements is possible until the people involved are aware that hearing loss is present and needs attention.

For some people who have undetected hearing loss, a gentle hint that their hearing may need to be checked is enough to increase awareness. For others, information about the high prevalence of hearing loss nationally to indicate that many people have it and it is not a shameful condition may be necessary. In addition, it can be helpful to provide information indicating that there is a variety of options for reducing any negative effects of hearing loss. Sometimes, making print information available for people to read (e.g., the Hearing Loss Association of America [HLAA] magazine), can alert them to awareness of their own potential hearing loss, and indicate steps to take.

Sometimes, the recognition that hearing loss affects those who are CPs as well as the PHL can induce someone to admit hearing loss and take positive steps to deal with it. For example, Joe may not be willing to admit to or deal with hearing loss for his own sake, but may do so in order to be helpful to his wife and kids.

Experience indicates there is a great need to provide information and training to professionals and staff who serve the public about hearing loss, its effects, and how to better communicate. Physical and mental health providers, educators, rehabilitation counselors, and similar will be working with PHLs who are either unaware or unwilling to discuss their hearing difficulties. Hearing loss may be preventing the person from accessing or properly using the services provided (e.g., unable to hear classroom lectures, unable to understand physician's recommendations) or being offered training for an unsuitable position (e.g., a control tower operator).

Sometimes, the unrecognized hearing loss causes or exacerbates other problems that the person is experiencing. For example, a PHL's high blood pressure may be related to the distress he or she experiences due to communication difficulties at home and at work. The marital problems discussed in therapy may be due in large part to difficulty understanding what a partner is saying.

Staff and professionals who know about hearing loss and its effects can detect the possibility of its presence and consider its influence on a client's life circumstances and suggest ways of assessing the hearing loss and procedures for accommodating it.

International Classification of Functioning, Disability and Health (ICF)

As discussed in Chapter 2, the International Classification of Functioning, Disability and Health (ICF) can be a helpful framework to understand and describe the consequences of hearing loss. In terms of the Brief ICF Core Sets (see Appendix) the following are categories that frequently are negatively impacted by hearing loss. *Attention* is a skill that can be eroded when a person tunes out of conversations due to difficulty understanding. *Structures of the brain* or neural connections can be lost due to disuse when certain auditory information is no longer registered in auditory areas of the cortex. *Family relationships* and *community life* are frequently altered by difficulties experienced by both the people who are talking and those who are trying to understand what is being said. *Education* and *employment* are often negatively affected by difficulty understanding what is being said in large listening environments in which there are multiple people speaking – often at the same time.

Considering these broad consequences, to adopt person-centered audiological rehabilitation (PCAR), the efforts of the clinician should be to make the PHL become aware of their hearing loss rather than offering them rehabilitation options at this phase.

Summary

When people are still in the preconscious stage of their hearing loss, they are unable to relate the inability to hear normally to other negative effects on their lives. Relationships at home or at work can be damaged by repeated communication difficulties that affect both the person who is speaking as well as the one who is listening. Inability to hear important environmental sounds can result in increased physical and psychological stress and the resulting negative emotional arousal that can trigger a variety of health problems. Untreated hearing loss can damage one's sense of acceptance by others, feelings of competence in one's work, and one's sense of influence or control over the physical and social environments. There are many ways of preventing or reducing the psychological, physical, and social problems related to hearing loss, including the use of electronic devices and adopting effective communication behavior tactics and strategies. However, the individual with hearing loss must first recognize the possibility of its presence and be open to considering its effects.

References

Alcock, C., 2015. It's not denial. It's observation. *Hearing Review*, 22(12), p. 16.

Cacioppo, J., 2003. The anatomy of loneliness. *Current Directions in Psychological Science*, 12(3), pp. 371–374.

Gagné, J., Southall, K., and Jennings, M., 2009. The psychological effects of social stigma: Applications to people with acquired hearing loss. In J. Montano and J. Spitzer (Eds.), *Advanced practice in adult audiological practice: International perspective*. San Diego, CA: Plural Publishing, Inc.

Horowitz, S., 2012. *The universal sense: How hearing shapes the mind*. New York, NY: Bloomsbury USA.

McCraty, R., 2001. *Science of the heart: Exploring the role of the heart in human performance*. Boulder Creek, CA: Institute of Heartmath.

McDonald, G. and Jensen-Campbell, L., 2011. *Social pain: Neuropsychological and health implications of loss and exclusion*. Washington, DC: American Psychological Association.

Trychin, S., 1990. *Why people don't acquire and/or wear hearing aids and other assistive listening devices*. Bethesda, MD: SHHH.

Trychin, S., 2013. *Living with hearing loss: Workbook (revised edition)*. Erie, PA: Self-published.

Trychin, S., 2014a. Mental health issues related to hearing loss. In J. Gournaris (Ed.), *Working with people with hearing loss: Mental health practitioner online training* [online]. Available from: http://registrations.dhs.state.mn.us/RegistrationCourses/HearingLoss/welcome_intro.html [Accessed 16 March 2016].

Trychin, S., 2014b. Peer support and consumer perspective. In J. J. Montano and J. B. Spitzer (Eds.), *Adult audiologic rehabilitation*, 2nd ed., pp. 517–534. San Diego, CA: Plural Publishing, Inc.

6

AWARENESS

Understanding and becoming aware of hearing loss

Sapna Mehta and Joseph Montano

Introduction

In the previous chapter, the pre-awareness phase of the patient journey with hearing loss was discussed and was illustrated by a number of scenarios. In this chapter, we will address the next phase – becoming aware of hearing loss. Some overlap exists between the pre-awareness and awareness phases of the journey as illustrated by the case examples provided. However, becoming aware and accepting the problem is a key step in the process of audiological rehabilitation.

A person's journey to awareness of hearing loss is influenced by a variety of internal and external factors that may influence both him/her and the significant communication partners (CPs). Some of these internal factors include an individual's perception of the stigma associated with hearing loss, coping strategies, and self-perceived limitations from a hearing problem. External factors relate to performance in various communication environments or situations, and the societal attitudes towards hearing loss. These factors may be influential long before the person has been evaluated by a clinician and a hearing loss has been diagnosed. The person with hearing loss (PHL) may begin to experience the effects of hearing loss before it is even suspected (Chia et al., 2007). A person's awareness of this loss will be affected by personal, emotional, social, and environmental factors. CPs will also be affected (Scarinci et al., 2008), and may in fact approach and accept the idea of a hearing loss even before the PHL. This chapter aims to explore what a PHL and his/her CPs experience as they become aware of a hearing loss, and the strategies they use to deal with the disability. We do not aim to determine factors that lead to help-seeking (see Knudsen et al., 2010), but rather aim to describe and explore the journey during the awareness phase. However, some attention will be given to studies that examine help-seeking behavior. This literature can contribute to our understanding of what individuals experience and consider during the period before they reach out for professional input.

Models of the patient journey

A person's experiences with hearing loss, termed the "patient journey," have been modeled as a continuum of phases (see Chapter 3). Manchaiah et al. (2011) describe seven phases of the patient journey through hearing loss, with the first two phases making up a significant portion of that journey, in which patients experience hearing loss before seeking further information or professional intervention. The first phase is one of pre-awareness, where people may experience the effects of hearing loss, but not consider it as contributing to any communication difficulties (Manchaiah et al., 2011) or quality of life issues that may be experienced (Chia et al., 2007). The second phase is one of awareness, in which people begin to suspect that their difficulties are related to a hearing loss, and may or may not begin to consider this a disability (Manchaiah et al., 2011). Subsequent phases lead to help-seeking and evaluation of proposed interventions. While this chapter will not discuss the later phases of the patient journey in detail, they will be considered as far as a person's expectations of these later stages may influence their experiences as they become aware of and accept the presence of a hearing loss.

Exploration of the awareness phase is important in understanding the overall journey for PHLs because they may spend a significant amount of time in this phase, in various states of readiness, as they begin to accept the existence of a hearing loss. Studies have found the awareness phase, in which a person realizes and may accept that he/she has a hearing loss, may last for years, on average 10 years (Davis et al., 2007), before a person decides to seek help or intervention. Therefore, a person's experiences during this time can be expected to play an important role in whether, and how, he/she approaches aural rehabilitation options, and how a person moves from becoming aware of a hearing problem, to deciding to do something about it.

The process of becoming aware of hearing loss may be based on the stages or the transtheoretical model of health behavior change, as described in Chapter 3. The awareness of hearing loss may occur anywhere throughout the pre-contemplation, contemplation, or preparation stages. A study conducted by Laplante-Lévesque and colleagues (2015) surveyed adults who failed an online hearing screening, and found that of the adults who failed the screening, and were thus aware of a hearing loss, most were in the contemplation stage or preparation stage, while a small percentage were considered to be in the pre-contemplation or action stages. Those adults who fell into the pre-contemplation stage identified with statements which characterized hearing loss as either not the individual's problem, a condition the individual may have but not problematic, as something to be avoided thinking about, or as something meant to be coped with, rather than changed. Statements that reflected feelings of acknowledging a hearing loss and a readiness to start to deal with it defined the contemplation stage. The preparation stage was defined by statements that indicated having started working on the hearing problem, but still seeking further help or willing to accept further help. It is worth noting that while all of these participants may be considered to be in the awareness phase, variation in acceptance of a hearing loss, and variation in readiness to consider seeking help or further information can be seen.

Awareness, acknowledgment, and acceptance

There are no set times for when a person with hearing loss becomes aware of its existence until the time when he/she acknowledges and accepts it. Awareness implies an experience that harkens a PHL to question why communication performance may have been difficult. While there may be multiple events of communication failure that could be considered part of awareness, it is not until the PHL acknowledges the possible contribution of hearing loss to those experiences that they can begin to accept it. Whatever it is they do about it, or however they choose to move forward, is deeply personal and individual. Some may choose to acknowledge the presence of hearing loss and do nothing about it; some may willingly act upon it by developing coping strategies and communication skills or seeking out hearing aids or aural rehabilitation. Still, some may acknowledge the presence of hearing loss and fight the need to improve their communication.

The effect of hearing loss on an individual's performance, in particular, the capacity to carry out hearing-related activities, and the ability to participate in communication and hearing-related social activities, may vary with the degree of hearing loss. However, the effect of hearing loss on a person will also be significantly influenced by various communication and personal factors (e.g., relationships, perception of the stigma associated with hearing loss, and coping strategies). The ways in which personal and environmental factors interact to influence the degree of activity limitations and participation restrictions, and the importance of these limitations to the individual with hearing loss, may help explain differences in self-perception due to hearing loss (Chang et al., 2009), and differences in readiness to accept its existence.

The following provides examples of how two individuals, both with a mild to moderate degree of hearing loss, related different experiences in becoming aware of a hearing loss, and different attitudes in their readiness to accept the hearing loss and understand its impact (names and specific details have been altered for all the examples in this chapter).

Example 1

Erica is a 75-year-old woman who recently retired. She generally did not believe she had much difficulty hearing, but, after retirement, as she started going out to restaurants with her friends more often, she noted that she had some trouble understanding conversations in noisy places. However, Erica's friends tended to be soft-spoken, so she was not sure that her communication difficulties were truly related to a hearing issue. She had also attended the theater more in the past few years, and had begun to seek out infrared headsets to use for a better listening experience. She felt that she did not always need to use these headsets in the theater, and sometimes felt they did not provide benefit in understanding the dialogue and listening to music. Again, she was unsure if her occasional problems hearing in some theaters were related to a hearing problem, or due to her location in the theater, acoustics, noise levels, or overall intelligibility of the actors themselves. However, Erica found another situation in which she did have some difficulty communicating, and took greater note due to its importance to her. Erica's grandson was a toddler who was beginning to string together words and enjoyed talking with his family. Erica saw him often, as her son's family lived in the same city, and they often dined together. She noticed that she was frequently having difficulty understanding what her grandson was saying, and found it effortful to engage with him, particularly at the dinner table, when there was a significant amount of competing noise and communication interference. Erica was again not sure if her difficulty understanding her grandson was due to a hearing problem, or due to the intelligibility of a toddler's speech; however, as understanding her grandson and participating in conversations with him was very important to Erica, she began to seriously contemplate the impact of a potential hearing problem on important relationships. She also began to reconsider other difficult listening situations, such as noisy restaurants, and theaters, in light of a potential hearing loss.

Erica was still unsure of her hearing ability, but tried to find other areas of her life that may be affected in order to gain a better grasp of the extent of the impact of a possible hearing loss. She found that in the majority of her day-to-day activities, she did not have significant difficulty hearing, and found that she was able to speak to her husband at home with no great difficulty, and use the telephone and watch television without a problem. However, when her son came over to her house, she noticed that he set the television to a lower volume than she preferred, and she had greater difficulty understanding the television at his chosen volume. This acted as another, almost quantifiable, indication to Erica that she may have a hearing problem, and reinforced her concerns about communicating with her grandson. After contemplating these various situations and weighing their importance, Erica began to consider a visit to her ear, nose, and throat physician, to inquire about hearing loss and find out what, if any, intervention may be available.

Example 2

Robert is a 68-year-old man who works in sales, has long workdays, and an active social life with his family and friends. Robert did not notice significant difficulty hearing compared to his peers. He did recognize that he occasionally had difficulty understanding conference calls, and missed some things at meetings, but did not feel that his difficulties were out of the ordinary, or that they hampered his ability to execute his work duties. Robert did not feel that he experienced any difficulty hearing when he was with his family, or when he was engaging in activities or gatherings with friends. He recognized that he may be gradually losing his hearing, and he suspected this was because both his parents had age-related hearing loss. However, he did not perceive his hearing loss as problematic and felt that his hearing ability was relatively normal compared to his peers.

Robert's wife, Betty, had experienced his hearing loss in a different way. She noticed that he had been having more difficulty hearing her speak around the house, that he had been increasing the volume on the television, and that it was necessary to repeat herself more often in order to accommodate his hearing difficulty. Betty also felt that he relied on her more to facilitate communication between friends and family at parties and other social events; she often repeated or rephrased a conversation for Robert so that he could avoid or correct misunderstandings. Betty was aware that he had a hearing problem, and saw how it may be affecting his communication socially and at home, but was also concerned about how it may be affecting his work. She expressed concern about how Robert's hearing may change in the future and increasingly interfere with his ability to communicate in all situations.

Betty encouraged him to see a doctor and have his hearing tested so they could better understand his hearing problems. She recommended he start to consider possible interventions and rehabilitation options. She began to point out instances where his communication breakdowns occurred in order to make him aware of the hearing difficulties that she observed. She was hopeful that by pointing out times when Robert experiences hardship, she would be able to convince him to seek help.

Robert ultimately agreed to go and see a doctor about his hearing. However, Robert still did not feel that his hearing loss was significant enough to warrant concern or action. He perceived his hearing loss as a normal part of life and thought that use of hearing aids would exaggerate his problem. While both Robert and Betty were aware of the hearing loss, they had different experiences and attitudes about it. Robert acknowledged his hearing loss, but did not perceive it as a limiting factor in his work or social lives, and thus did not think he needed to take any action. Betty, on the other hand, accepted his hearing loss and felt it had been having an impact on his communication ability in all situations. Any movement Robert made towards addressing his hearing loss was influenced by his wife, and he himself was not yet ready to take steps to address a hearing problem.

Communication partners

As discussed in Chapter 4, CPs are influential in the help-seeking behaviors of people with hearing loss, and it is important to consider their journey. CPs may enter the awareness stage before or in tandem with the PHL; regardless, they will likely experience this stage differently. In the example provided above, Betty can be seen to experience activity limitations in how she is able to communicate with Robert at home; she is no longer able to casually speak to him while washing the dishes or when the television is on in the background without first getting his attention. She also experiences participation limitations due to her perception that Robert relies on her during social interactions for correcting communication breakdowns, causing her to feel that she cannot leave him alone for long at social gatherings. Betty's experiences during her awareness stage are also influenced by environmental factors such as the noisy nature of the listening environments she is often in with Robert, and by personal factors such as her own perceptions of the stigma associated with hearing difficulties and her desire to avoid the application of these negative associations to her husband.

Awareness of hearing changes

The remainder of this chapter will examine some of the factors that may affect the experiences of a PHL and his/her CPs as they become aware of a hearing problem. Self-perceived hearing constraints and perception of communication difficulties have been found to be related to help-seeking behavior and acceptance of interventions (Humes et al., 2003; Laplante-Lévesque et al., 2013), and therefore may also play a role during the awareness phase of hearing loss, as the examples above demonstrate.

Another factor that plays a role in how a person begins to suspect a hearing problem is the recognition of changes in hearing ability that are not related to communication (see Chapter 5). For example, the loss of the ability to hear environmental sounds, or the onset of tinnitus, may prompt a person to become aware of a possible hearing loss. The following are examples of people who began to suspect hearing loss due to non-communication related changes:

Example 3

Helen is a 60-year-old woman who enjoys bird-watching, and is often accompanied by her friend, James, in this activity. Helen generally had no difficulties hearing, although she occasionally noticed that she had trouble understanding some of her students when they were speaking quickly among themselves in her classroom. Helen began to notice that when she would go bird-watching with James, her friend would hear birdcalls that Helen would miss. Helen began to suspect that she might be losing her hearing. After a few months of considering what to do about it, she decided to have her hearing tested. Her motivation is concern that a hearing loss may interfere with her enjoyment of bird-watching.

Example 4

John is a musician and began noticing tinnitus when he was in college. As his tinnitus was constant and bothersome, he visited his doctor and was ultimately recommended to have a hearing test. John's audiogram revealed a hearing loss. He was not surprised by this finding due to his perception of tinnitus, and his history of working around loud music. However, John had felt extremely stressed during the test, and was still unsure if it was an accurate representation of his hearing sensitivity. John put off returning for tests to monitor his hearing due to his distrust of their accuracy, and due to his expectations that any clinician conducting the test would not understand that he was not concerned about his hearing ability, but rather, his tinnitus. John knew that he had a hearing loss, but he did not feel this was his primary concern. He felt that he would not get the help he sought for his tinnitus by thinking about his hearing. Over a few years, John learned to cope with tinnitus at home by using a sound machine to act as a tinnitus masker. He continued to do research on tinnitus therapies and management options on his own, as he continued to feel bothered by tinnitus. He did not feel that he needed to deal with his hearing loss during this time, since he did not perceive it to be a problem. However, when his tinnitus changed and became louder in one ear, he became concerned about a medical problem and revisited the doctor. He was again asked to have a hearing test, which he did, though somewhat reluctantly. He continued to express distrust of the hearing test, and noted that he already knew he had a hearing loss. When tinnitus management options were discussed with him by the clinician and physician, including the possibility of managing his hearing loss, John decided that he would rather continue to find a way to cope with tinnitus on his own, as he still felt that he could not trust his clinicians to understand his problem.

The effect of perception of and trust in health professionals

As can be seen from the example above, perceptions and expectations of the clinicians who deal with hearing loss can affect a patient's experiences during the awareness phase of their journey. Trust of health professionals and expectations of the diagnostic and aural rehabilitation processes (see Chapters 8 and 9) may be based on preconceived ideas, word-of-mouth experiences of friends and family, or direct experiences with health professionals. This can influence how a PHL ultimately accepts and deals with his/her hearing loss once aware of its existence (Meyer and Hickson, 2012). Studies that have examined factors which affect the decision to move forward with hearing aids do not directly address the awareness phase of a person's journey with hearing loss; however, these studies can be instructive in comprehending what people contemplate during the awareness phase when deciding whether or not to seek help. Garstecki and Erler (1998) and Kochkin (2007) found that expectations about professional trustworthiness, cost of hearing aids, perception about difficulty of use of hearing aids, and poor expected benefit, deterred some people with hearing loss from deciding to seek professional help. Therefore, expectations of the aural rehabilitation process may play a role in how people decide whether they should take action to address a hearing loss.

Stigma and perceived stigma of hearing loss

Expectations about how others may perceive an acknowledged hearing loss is an important contributing factor for many during the awareness process. PHLs and their CPs may be influenced by what they perceive are the beliefs of others. In some societies, hearing loss may be associated with negative traits, such as reduced mental capacity, and frailty due to aging, which are attributed to the PHL in a process called stigmatization (Gagné et al., 2009). The stigmatization of hearing loss in an individual's community, or his/her perception of the stigma in society can influence how a person and his/her CP choose to approach a hearing loss. The PHL and CP may be aware of the stigma associated with hearing loss, and may feel that they are likely to have to confront people who hold the stigma to be true once the disability becomes observable. Furthermore, the PHL may self-stigmatize and believe the associated negative personal characteristics, as too, the CPs may also believe in these negative stereotypes (Gagné et al., 2009). A person who self-stigmatizes, or who recognizes that close CPs and other community members believe in the negative stereotypes of PHLs, may experience their awareness process in a variety of ways. They may acknowledge hearing difficulties, but attribute these difficulties to environmental and external factors, such as excessive background noise, effectively separating the hearing difficulty from a self-identity. On the other hand, a person who is aware of a hearing loss may avoid difficult listening environments and reduce participation in activities that require significant communication in order to make the hearing problem less conspicuous, so that they may avoid any stigmatizing effects. However, a person may also acknowledge a hearing loss, and be aware and concerned about the stigmatization of hearing loss, but may ultimately decide that the efforts and personal and social costs required to conceal the hearing loss outweigh the potential and perceived costs of seeking help for a hearing problem (Gagné et al., 2009). The following examples demonstrate how individuals with hearing loss may experience and cope with the stigmatizing effect of hearing loss in different ways as they become aware of and acknowledge a hearing loss.

Example 5

Jack is a retired grandfather with hearing loss who lives near his children and grandchildren and notices difficulty hearing all of them, but especially his grandchildren. His family is aware of his hearing difficulty, but they find it exasperating to have to repeat themselves when speaking to him. Jack noticed that his grandchildren avoid spending too much time with him and do not share news about their school lives with him. He also noticed that his children frequently sigh or express frustration when they are speaking to him, and they no longer come to him for advice. Jack feels guilty that he is the cause of their frustration, and angered that his children and grandchildren do not do more to help ease communication and include him in their lives. Therefore, while Jack still spends time at his children's homes, he avoids participating in conversations and continues to feel left out of his family.

Example 6

Sally is a project manager at a large company. She noticed difficulty hearing her project team members in meetings, and suspected that she may have a hearing loss because no one else in these meetings seemed have any difficulty understanding these conversations. However, Sally does not want to have her hearing checked because she thinks this will ultimately lead to hearing aids, which she does not want to wear. She is worried that people who might notice her hearing aids would think that she may not be capable of leading her team, or that attention on the hearing aids would detract from her accomplishments at her job. Sally decides instead to manage her difficult listening situation by moving the meetings to a smaller conference room, and enforcing a more structured format, so that people in the meetings speak in turn, and speaking all at once is discouraged. These changes allow her to more easily understand what is said in meetings, while still allowing her to conceal her hearing difficulty from her coworkers.

As can be seen from the examples above, stigma associated with hearing loss can strongly influence how individuals cope with their awareness of a hearing problem. Jack's case demonstrates that social attitudes towards hearing loss can have an impact on how people feel about their own hearing loss, and that avoidance of difficult listening situations can be a coping strategy for people who wish to distance themselves from negative characteristics assigned to PHLs. Sally's case shows that some individuals may opt to use positive coping strategies when dealing with hearing loss, by taking action to correct a difficult listening environment, even though they may still feel they have to deal with the stigma associated with hearing loss.

Therefore, while a person may have greater awareness and acceptance of hearing loss if they notice that hearing and communication difficulties are limiting their activities and participation in important social events or relationships, perceived stigma of hearing loss is also an important factor in how a person copes with hearing loss. As the examples in this chapter demonstrate, the belief that hearing loss is associated with negative personal characteristics can influence a person to attempt to conceal the loss and deny it as problematic, or avoid difficult interactions. It is also possible that an individual will internalize the stigma, and avoid considering that communication problems may be due to a hearing loss. Perceived societal attitudes towards hearing loss can have a significant impact on the strategies a person uses to cope with a hearing loss, and on their journey from awareness to action.

Summary

It is apparent that PHLs and their CPs face a complex interaction of personal and societal beliefs about hearing loss, and limitations in activities and social engagement or participation. These influencing factors may help to explain why PHLs continue in the awareness phase for many years before deciding to seek help, and it may help explain the diversity of experiences people have as they become aware of a hearing loss. It is important for clinicians, PHLs, and their CPs to better understand this part of the patient journey so that meaningful help-seeking behavior can be encouraged.

References

Chang, H., Ho, C., and Chou, P., 2009. The factors associated with a self-perceived hearing handicap in elderly people with hearing impairment – results from a community-based study. *Ear and Hearing*, 30(5), pp. 576–583.

Chia, E., Wang, J., Rochtchina, E., Cumming, R., Newall, P., and Mitchell, P., 2007. Hearing impairment and health-related quality of life: The Blue Mountains hearing study. *Ear and Hearing*, 28(2), pp. 187–195.

Davis, A., Smith, P., Ferguson, M., Stephens, D., and Gianopoulos, I., 2007. Acceptability, benefit and costs of early screening for hearing disability: A study of potential screening tests and models. *Health Technology Assessment*, 11(42), pp. 1–294.

Gagné, J.-P., Southall, K., and Jennings, M., 2009. The psychological effects of social stigma: Applications to people with an acquired hearing loss. In J.J. Montano and J.B. Spitzer (Eds.), *Adult Audiologic Rehabilitation* (pp. 63–91). San Diego, CA: Plural Publishing, Inc.

Garstecki, D. and Erler, S., 1998. Hearing loss, control, and demographic factors influencing hearing aid use among older adults. *Journal of Speech, Language, and Hearing Research*, 41(3), pp. 527–537.

Humes, L., Wilson, D., and Humes, A., 2003. Examination of differences between successful and unsuccessful elderly hearing aid candidates matched for age, hearing loss and gender. *International Journal of Audiology*, 42(7), pp. 432–441.

Knudsen, L., Öberg, M., Nielsen, C., Naylor, G., and Kramer, S., 2010. Factors influencing help seeking, hearing aid uptake, hearing aid use and satisfaction with hearing aids: A review of the literature. *Trends in Amplification*, 14(3), pp. 127–154.

Kochkin, S., 2007. MarkeTrak VII: Obstacles to adult non-user adoption of hearing aids. *The Hearing Journal*, 60(4), pp. 24–50.

Laplante-Lévesque, A., Hickson, L., and Worrall, L., 2013. Stages of change in adults with acquired hearing impairment seeking help for the first time: Application of the transtheoretical model in audiologic rehabilitation. *Ear and Hearing*, 34(4), pp. 447–457.

Laplante-Lévesque, A., Brännström, K., Ingo, E., Andersson, G., and Lunner, T., 2015. Stages of change in adults who have failed an online hearing screening. *Ear and Hearing*, 36(1), pp. 92–101.

Manchaiah, V., Stephens, D., and Meredith, R., 2011. The patient journey of adults with hearing impairment: The patients' views. *Clinical Otolaryngology*, 36(3), pp. 227–234.

Meyer, C. and Hickson, L., 2012. What factors influence help-seeking for hearing impairment and hearing aid adoption in older adults? *International Journal of Audiology*, 51(2), pp. 66–74.

Scarinci, N., Worrall, L., and Hickson, L., 2008. The effect of hearing impairment in older people on the spouse. *International Journal of Audiology*, 47(3), pp. 141–151.

7

MOVEMENT

Making steps to seek information, help, and intervention

Lindsey E. Jorgensen, Margaret Nowak, and Patricia McCarthy

Introduction

After becoming aware of hearing loss and its consequences, some people may choose to do something about the problem. This chapter focuses on the process of seeking information and help. It is important to recognize that the acceptance of hearing loss must happen before the person with hearing loss (PHL) starts to seek information and explore options (i.e., movement phase) to address consequences of hearing loss. However, sometimes the PHL may also engage in the movement phase due to external factors such as influence of communication partners (CPs). We start with the following illustration to demonstrate the complexity of this phase:

> Mr. Walker is a 64-year-old retired police officer and Vietnam veteran. He first experienced difficulty in communicating with his wife and friends at their weekly lunch gatherings. At the urging of his wife, he searched the Internet for the number of the local Veterans Affairs Medical Center and consulted the Internet for information on hearing loss. However, Mr. Walker postponed calling the Veterans Affairs to make an appointment to seek professional help and continued to live with the detrimental social and personal effects of his hearing loss for almost a decade. About nine years later, his compromised ability to hear his three grandchildren coupled with his wife's frustration led him finally to make an appointment for a hearing aid evaluation. Mr. Walker's story begs the question: What happens between the moments an individual notices he/she has a hearing loss and his/her decision to seek professional help?

The patient journey to seek help for hearing loss is a complex and often long process. The term "patient journey" is used to describe the milestones and experiences an individual endures during the disease course and treatment (Ida Institute, 2009). A person with hearing loss typically will go through various experiences and steps before, during, and after he/she becomes aware of hearing loss. As detailed in Chapters 1 and 3, the seven phases of the patient journey include: (1) Pre-awareness, (2) Awareness, (3) Movement, (4) Diagnostics, (5) Rehabilitation, (6) Self-evaluation, and (7) Resolution. It is crucial for healthcare professionals to recognize the entire patient journey to better understand how individuals can successfully make steps towards movement and action. In this chapter, we examine that portion of the patient journey that involves movement towards seeking information, help, and intervention for hearing loss.

Public health perspective/concern

The widespread prevalence of hearing loss is surprising to many people, perhaps because it is often considered an "invisible disability." Yet, the World Health Organization (WHO) estimates that one-third of people over 65 years old, or about 328 million adults worldwide, are affected by disabling hearing loss (e.g., greater than 40 dB in the better hearing ear) (World Health Organization, 2015). As the global population ages, there is a growing need for affordable and accessible hearing healthcare. Less than 20 percent of individuals with hearing loss who need intervention actually seek help, thus making it a major public health concern (Donahue et al., 2010). Additionally, the societal and personal consequences of undetected and untreated hearing loss have become of concern to government and public policy making bodies across the globe (see Chapter 1).

The growing need for audiologic rehabilitation in the aging population is a public health concern particularly for people whose age, race, ethnicity, gender, occupation, or health status leads to an increased risk of hearing loss. Consequently, increasing the adoption rate of hearing aid usage has been a major public health focus of the twenty-first century and the World Health Organization. However, few accessible low-cost rehabilitation options currently exist. As such, financial obstacles to obtaining hearing aids are primary reasons individuals with hearing loss do not seek professional help across the globe. Yet as the global population ages, there is an increasing need for affordable and accessible hearing healthcare.

Financial concerns continue to be a negative factor in the hearing rehabilitation process in many countries (e.g., the United States and India); access to healthcare in general is a major political and public policy issue. Additionally, many third-party payers do not provide coverage for hearing aids and government subsidies are not currently available. It should be noted that cost is not likely to be a factor in countries wherein hearing aids and rehabilitation are part of the national healthcare service and individuals are not charged.

For those who can afford hearing aids, consumer access to obtain hearing healthcare help can be challenging. Multiple professionals and sources of information (e.g., primary care physicians, audiologists, hearing aid specialists, otolaryngologists, internet) can be confusing, contradictory, and discouraging to consumers with hearing loss and their families. As such, individuals may remain in the awareness phase because movement to the action stage is a daunting challenge.

Contemporary healthcare systems encourage screening for hearing loss for every patient using tools such as the Hearing Handicap Inventory for the Elderly (HHIE) questionnaire. If an individual does not pass the screening, the physician should provide education, counseling, and a referral. However, Kochkin (2007) reported that merely 15 percent of individuals over 65 years old are screened for hearing loss annually by their primary care physician. Consequently, even when adults at risk for hearing loss are seen by their primary care physicians, hearing loss is likely not addressed thus contributing to delay in diagnosis and rehabilitation.

From a public health perspective, individuals who are in the pre-awareness or awareness phases of their journey towards hearing diagnosis and rehabilitation may face societal and institutional obstacles that slow or delay their movement towards action. Societal costs of untreated hearing loss are continuing to mount on a global basis. In fact, hearing loss was ranked 15th among the leading causes of burden of disease in 2004 but will rise to 7th by 2030 (World Health Organization, 2008). Clearly, with the rising burden of hearing loss on individuals and their families, society must embrace the gravity of this public policy crisis and develop improved mechanisms for improving access to diagnosis and rehabilitation.

Steps towards movement

As mentioned in Chapter 3, the patient journey towards rehabilitation is not viewed as a linear, step-wise progression; however, it is important that a PHL is first aware and accepting of their hearing loss before they enter the movement phase. Taking action to deal with hearing loss is dependent on attitude/acceptance, i.e., does the individual have a favorable attitude towards hearing aids and the rehabilitation process? If so, he/she is more likely to engage in the process. Are family members and/or CP supportive of the process? If yes, again the individual is more likely to move from the awareness to the diagnostic phase. Finally, do societal and cultural norms support hearing aids and hearing rehabilitation? Alternatively, are there pervasive societal norms that contribute to negative connotations about hearing aids? Modern society, while making strides, still condones the hearing aid stigma (see Chapter 1).

Conventional wisdom continues to perpetrate negative attitudes that associate hearing aids with aging and dementia. As an individual contemplates a move towards seeking information and intervention, negative attitudes, lack of family support, and/or negative cultural norms can undermine the individual's journey by delaying treatment. The odds of an individual taking action when faced with these attitudes are very small; however, the PHL can still overcome societal and individual barriers to seek hearing help.

The perspectives of the PHL, CPs, and healthcare providers can all play a role in the PHL's decision to make steps towards movement. During the movement phase, the PHL may seek information about hearing loss from a primary care physician, family, friends, internet, newspaper, and/or magazine advertisements. The PHL may express their concerns and expectations about hearing loss solutions to those around them in order to obtain insight on how to proceed. If a PHL does not perceive his/her hearing loss as severe enough to warrant treatment, he/she may look for validation from others that they are justified to not seek help. On the other hand, a PHL will be more likely to commit to rehabilitation if he/she believes life and relationships will improve as a result (Schum, 2014). After obtaining information about hearing loss, the PHL may decide that the potential benefits of intervention exceed the perceived costs (e.g., financial, stigma, time, effort). At that point, the PHL may arrange a referral to a hearing healthcare professional or search for providers in the area in order to take steps towards diagnosis and intervention.

Contemporary healthcare consumerism and financial incentives may also play a large role in an individual's willingness to make a decision. The vast amount of information available on the internet as well as the multiple entry points to the hearing healthcare system may cause a PHL to remain stagnant in the movement phase. Individuals may continue to price shop and compare providers for some time before they decide when and where they will go to seek help for their hearing loss (Schum, 2014). As such, the actions that take place during the movement phase are largely dependent on the PHL and CP's perspectives in addition to influential internal and external factors.

Factors influencing movement towards seeking help

Despite reports that hearing loss is the third most prevalent chronic health conditions facing older adults, self-report of hearing loss often relates poorly to results of clinically measured hearing loss. This suggests that people can be poor reporters of the presence or degree of their hearing loss. Further, hearing testing alone is not a good predictor of the desire to pursue amplification or other communication strategies. The motivation to seek information from a hearing healthcare provider, however, does not correlate with the individual's desire to pursue a hearing aid solution for a disabling condition (Clausen and Pryce, 2012). Some individuals may be seen for a hearing evaluation only to appease family members and/or CPs; they have little intrinsic desire to pursue rehabilitation. Others may be seeking education, reassurance, or support for their condition.

Those who do perceive a hearing problem typically are more willing to seek assistance for the problem. Based on self-report alone, Palmer and colleagues (2009) reported a significant correlation between those who self-report hearing difficulties and obtain hearing aids. However, individuals who schedule hearing evaluations tend to fall into one of two groups: (1) those who acknowledge a hearing problem and are seeking a solution; and (2) those who do not believe they have a problem and want confirmation of normal auditory ability. As such, action in the form of undergoing a hearing evaluation does not predict further help-seeking action; therefore, other motivational factors must influence.

The motivation to seek hearing healthcare varies from person to person with each individual experiencing a different journey. The clear movement from pre-awareness and awareness to movement and diagnosis phases is not predictable among adults with hearing loss. It is interesting that although treatment of other sensory systems (like vision problems) is seen as commonplace, seeking treatment for hearing loss appears to involve more pre-awareness and awareness time. Once the PHL reaches acceptance, however, it is likely that he/she will seek some form of assistance. This section we will discuss a few of those factors which may influence a person's hearing health-seeking behavior.

There are myriad demographic factors prompting a PHL's decision to pursue a solution to his/her hearing problems including age, gender, social life, living arrangements, level of education, and age at onset of hearing loss. While little research on the impact of age and gender on hearing healthcare-seeking behaviors exist, other areas of medical care have noted a significant difference between the rates at which men seek assistance as compared with women (Li et al., 2007). Age may also significantly change a person's health-seeking behavior, as older adults are less likely to seek healthcare as early as younger adults are.

Socioeconomic status has been suggested to have a significant influence on health-seeking behavior; however, the link is thought to be related to general health knowledge. In general, those with lower household incomes are less likely to seek healthcare from a qualified professional (Ahmed et al., 2005) and those with higher socioeconomic status are more likely to seek assistance given their financial means and broader knowledge about healthcare. This trend may not hold up in hearing healthcare; people with higher socioeconomic status were found to be less likely to self-report hearing difficulty (Benova et al., 2015). This finding may reflect the ongoing hearing loss stigma that cuts across socioeconomic groups.

The age of onset of hearing loss, rapidity of degradation, and etiology may also play a significant role in whether an individual seeks hearing care. Individuals with sudden hearing loss or onset at an early age are more likely to seek care from a hearing healthcare professional. This is likely due to the sudden, deleterious impact on a person's communication and lifestyle. Individuals with gradual progressive hearing loss may adapt over time and not recognize the incipient onset and deleterious effects on communication and lifestyle.

It is likely that personality traits may influence an individual to seek assistance and move into the action stage earlier. The role of personality has been explored to determine its role in the hearing loss journey, particularly in the area of hearing aid uptake. However, little research has investigated the role of personality in hearing healthcare seeking and acceptance behavior.

The presence of co-morbidities may influence hearing health-seeking behaviors. PHLs with other significant diagnoses may be less likely to seek professional preventative or specialty services. Patients experiencing multiple and/or significant health conditions may prioritize their health conditions. Given that hearing loss is not life threatening, it may be given a lower status by individuals battling serious diseases/disorders. As an individual contemplates a move towards seeking information and intervention, negative attitudes, lack of family support, and/or negative cultural norms can undermine the individual's journey by delaying treatment. The odds of an individual taking action when faced with these attitudes are very small; however, the PHL can still overcome societal and individual barriers to seek hearing help.

An individual's social life, living arrangement, recreational activities, and other environmental factors can contribute to his/her movement towards action. Personal acknowledgment of the activity and participation restrictions and limitations imposed by hearing loss appear to influence motivation to take action. The individual who is active in the community, has extensive communication demands, and/or engages in various social activities may be more likely to seek information and assistance as he/she experiences limitations and participation restrictions. While Mr. Walker recognized his hearing difficulties on some level, he did not acknowledge the effects of hearing loss on his quality of life. A person must see a positive cost/benefit of rehabilitation in order to move towards action. Good external support and a willingness to put forth the effort needed to succeed with hearing technology are essential for a PHL to seek hearing healthcare and perceive benefit from rehabilitation.

Influence of family and primary health providers

While denial of a hearing problem remains a common thread of internal resistance to hearing heathcare, family members and/or CPs often notice the problem much earlier and commonly are instigators of audiologic appointments. As such, an individual in the pre-awareness and awareness phases may be pushed to take action in the form of a hearing assessment only to appease others. At this point in the journey, the influence of family members and other CPs can only reach so far. Mr. Walker, as described above, obtained information about where to seek information and help for hearing loss at the behest of his wife. However, it still took almost a decade for him to move into the action stage.

Many people are persuaded by a family member to consult a doctor regarding hearing loss so the primary care physician is often the first professional seen in the individual's hearing loss journey. This entry into the action phase can enable an individual to move towards the action stage or can enable him/her to remain in the pre-awareness phase. PHLs often feel uncertain about the potential benefit of audiological management but likely will respect the advice of their primary care physician. It is well documented that the most important social influence for the decision to adopt hearing aids is the family physician. In fact, patients are eight times more likely to purchase hearing assistive technology if their physician has recommended it yet few primary care physicians routinely check or refer for hearing difficulties (Jorgensen et al., 2014). Furthermore, often physicians may tell them that they did not need hearing aids or that hearing aids would not help them. Furthermore, physicians may not be up-to-date on current hearing aid technology and may give outdated information thus discouraging patients from seeking care from a qualified hearing healthcare professional. An individual may be swayed to seek hearing assistance sooner or avoid it when needed based on physician recommendations. Yet, the validity of the recommendation for rehabilitative follow-up may be questionable thus delaying the individual's journey towards rehabilitative action.

Once a person has decided to pursue a consultation with a hearing healthcare provider, there are external factors that can facilitate or undermine action including the referral pathway. Hickson et al. (1999) found that self-motivation to seek healthcare is associated with satisfaction with the hearing device. This latter report reinforces the need for providing information and education about the value of the rehabilitation process as the PHL moves towards the action phase.

The provider's qualifications and expertise can significantly influence success with hearing technology and communication strategies. This part of the journey often contributes to confusion and a stalling at the pre-awareness and awareness phases. The multiple levels of providers who offer hearing healthcare are difficult for the consumer to untangle and may lead to inaction. Mr. Walker knew he could seek the services of a qualified audiologist at the Veterans Affairs Medical Center. However, the pathway is not always so clear. Media advertisements can contribute to the confusion as full-page newspaper ads for hearing aids make unverifiable claims and offer "free services." Thus, even the individual who is ready to move from the pre-awareness to the action phase may be stymied as to how to even enter the hearing healthcare system. Consequently, confusion in provider qualifications and navigating the healthcare system may decrease motivation and delay the journey towards improved communication.

Person-centered audiologic rehabilitation

There is a well-accepted maxim that "there is an average 7–10 year lapse between the time an adult notices a hearing loss and the time that they actually do something about it" which bears further examination. This average does not tell the whole story and can be misleading. Schum (2014) reported a bi-modal pattern in describing when people take action with their hearing loss. Results showed that a large percentage of individuals actually do initiate action within the first 1–2 years of noticing hearing problems. However, that number steadily decreased over the next seven years; as the years of living with hearing loss accrued, the likelihood of seeking assistance decreased. The bi-modal pattern also showed another bump at the ten-year mark when the largest percentage actually pursued help for their hearing loss. In other words, one group of adults was ready to seek assistance for their hearing problems within the first few years of noticing a problem while the other group waited nearly a decade before seeking help. Recall Mr. Walker, the patient described above, who waited for almost a decade before making an appointment for a hearing aid evaluation, clearly placing him in the second group described by Schum (2014).

It is critical that hearing health providers understand the implications of this bi-modal behavior pattern because of the implications for rehabilitation.

During the pre-awareness and awareness phases, individuals will continue to experience the compounding negative effects of untreated hearing loss on personal, family, and societal levels. Yet, the rehabilitative needs of an adult who has identified hearing difficulties within the past 1–2 years are vastly different from the needs of an individual who has been coping and struggling with hearing loss for a decade.

Contemporary hearing rehabilitation of adults with acquired hearing loss is person-centered and outcome driven. As detailed in Chapter 2, the World Health Organization's (WHO) International Classification of Functioning, Disability and Health (ICF) is a contemporary framework that examines health outcomes in regards to health and functioning (World Health Organization, 2001). This model emphasizes the complex interaction of body function and structure (e.g., motivation, auditory perception), activities (e.g., listening), participation (e.g., interpersonal interactions), and environmental factors (e.g., attitudes of immediate family, health professionals). However, ultimately, outcomes are significantly influenced by the initial part of the individual's journey. Treatment planning, involving the individual, family members, and/or communication partners, must reflect on how the individual got to the action stage in order to plan for successful outcomes. Ignoring that part of the journey belies the expectations, attitudes, experiences, and other factors that can undermine the process.

For individuals who are aware of their hearing loss, but are to seek intervention (i.e., awareness phase), the healthcare provider plays a key role in providing relevant information, support, and guidance. Comprehensive case-history taking and use of self-report tools are essential to working with these individuals. Self-report tools, assessing multiple domains, provide extensive, valuable information about the individual's activity and participation restrictions as well as social and emotional effects of hearing loss. A unique self-assessment questionnaire developed by Saunders and colleagues (2012) uses the stages of change model to quantify perceived severity, susceptibility, and patient movement towards action. Individuals in this stage will need counseling focused on the psychological, social, emotional, and occupational effects of hearing loss, the benefits of amplification and rehabilitation, realistic expectations, and his/her personal goals. The hearing care provider can play a critical role in arming the individual with the information needed for him/her to move towards making an action plan. Indeed, the hearing care provider's goal is to guide the individual's movement towards action.

For individuals who have spent extensive time in the pre-awareness and awareness phases, the rehabilitative challenges may be more daunting. Indeed, psychosocial health declines with more severe hearing loss (Donahue et al., 2010). Individuals who adopt hearing aids earlier on may demonstrate better outcomes with amplification. Similarly, as hearing loss becomes more severe over time, the rehabilitation process gets more complex and may require more time and intensity. These individuals, in conjunction with family and/or CPs, will need individualized plans focused on coping and communication strategies, amplification and bi-sensory communication in addition to psychosocial counseling and development of realistic expectations. Self-assessment tools, patient education materials, and counseling will be essential for individuals who have lived with untreated hearing loss for over a decade.

Summary

The individual's journey from the pre-awareness phase to seeking information, help, and intervention with his/her hearing loss is highly variable and subject to myriad intrinsic and extrinsic factors. In the movement phase, the PHL tends to seek input and information about hearing loss from a primary care physician, family, friends, internet, newspaper, and/or magazine advertisements before taking steps to seek diagnosis and intervention. It is the complex interaction of many perspectives, experiences, and factors that prompts people to seek help for their hearing loss. There is large variability in the time and actions (linear or not) it takes for an individual to recognize hearing loss and ultimately to take action, and this will have an influence on rehabilitative outcome. Individuals may have multiple entry points to the hearing healthcare system and may be at different stages in their journey, but all share a common goal, i.e., improved communication. Mr. Walker was able to navigate his way towards mitigating the impact of hearing loss on his communication ability. There were many influences on his path towards acceptance and help – some facilitating and some inhibiting his journey. These influences vary among individuals, but all significantly influence their hearing healthcare-seeking behavior.

References

Ahmed, S., Tomson, G., Petzold, M., and Kabir, Z., 2005. Socioeconomic status overrides age and gender in determining health-seeking behavior in rural Bangladesh. *Bulletin of the World Health Organization*, 83, pp. 109–117.

Benova, L., Grundy, E., and Ploubidis, G., 2015. Socioeconomic position and health-seeking behavior for hearing loss among older adults in England. *Journals of Gerontology: Series B, Gerontological Society of America*, 70(3), pp. 443–452.

Claesen, E. and Pryce, H., 2012. An exploration of the perspective of help-seekers prescribed hearing aids. *Primary Health Care Research and Development*, 13(3), pp. 279–284.

Donahue, A., Dubno, J., and Beck, L., 2010. Accessible and affordable hearing health care for adults with mild to moderate hearing loss. *Ear and Hearing*, 31, pp. 2–6.

Hickson, L., Timm, M., and Worrall, L., 1999. Hearing aid fitting: Outcomes for older adults. *Australian Journal of Audiology*, 21, pp. 9–21.

Ida Institute, 2009. A possible patient journey. *Ida Institute* [online]. Available at: http://idainstitute.com/toolbox/ci_resources/self_development/get_started/patient_journey/ [Accessed on 16 March 2016].

Jorgensen, L., Palmer, C., and Fischer, G., 2014. Evaluation of hearing status at the time of dementia diagnosis. *Audiology Today*, 26(1), pp. 38–42.

Kochkin, S., 2007. MarkeTrak VII: Obstacles to adult non-user adoption of hearing aids. *The Hearing Journal*, 60(4), pp. 27–43.

Li, Y., Cai, X., Glance, L., and Mukamel, D., 2007. Gender differences in healthcare-seeking behavior for urinary incontinence and the impact of socioeconomic status: A study of the Medicare managed care population. *Medical Care*, 45(11), pp. 1116–1122.

Palmer, C., Solodar, H., Hurley, W., Byrne, D., and Williams, K., 2009. Self-perception of hearing ability as a strong predictor of hearing aid purchase. *Journal of the American Academy of Audiology*, 20(6), pp. 341–347.

Saunders, G., Chisolm, T., and Wallhagen, M., 2012. Older adults and hearing help-seeking behaviors. *American Journal of Audiology*, 21(2), pp. 331–337.

Schum, D., 2014. The emergence of hearing loss in adult patient. *Audiology Online* [online]. Available at: www.audiologyonline.com/articles/emergence-hearing-loss-in-adult-765 [Accessed on 16 March 2016].

World Health Organization, 2001. *International Classification of Functioning, Disability and Health (ICF)*. Geneva, Switzerland: World Health Organization.

World Health Organization, 2008. The burden of disease: 2004 update. *World Health Organization* [online]. Available at: www.who.int/healthinfo/global_burden_disease/GBD_report_2004update_full.pdf [Accessed on 16 March 2016].

World Health Organization, 2015. Deafness and hearing loss. *World Health Organization* [online]. Available at: www.who.int/mediacentre/factsheets/fs300/en/ [Accessed on 16 March 2016].

8

EVALUATION AND DIAGNOSIS

Understanding, communication, and shared decision making

Fei Zhao, Calum Delaney, and Wenlong Xiong

Introduction

As described in the previous chapters, after becoming aware of hearing loss and hav-ing taken action to seek information, the person with hearing loss (PHL) may decide to start the journey of consultation and possible intervention with hearing health-care professionals. As a part of this journey, audiological services and procedures provide an evaluation of hearing and related difficulties, followed by a diagnosis and the development of a plan for the management of the difficulties. The main purpose of this is to facilitate improved communication in PHLs, which will in turn improve health-related quality of life (HRQoL) by reducing the psychological, social, and emotional effects of hearing loss (Gagné et al., 2009). According to the modern audiological rehabilitation concept developed on the basis of the World Health Organization's (WHO) International Classification of Functioning, Disability and Health (ICF; World Health Organization, 2001), using the biopsychosocial model, audiological services are expected to go beyond the traditional approach in order to adopt a more holistic, person-centered orientation in hearing healthcare. Decisions in the management of hearing loss should not only consider functional hearing deficits, but also the effects on the psychological, social, and socio-economic status of the person, as well as the overall effect on HRQoL (Gagné et al., 2009). Using a biopsychosocial approach to implement audiological management, it is impor-tant for hearing health professionals (HHPs) to adopt person-centered audiological rehabilitation (PCAR) by using effective patient-centered communication, together with a consideration of patients' values and the contributions they are able to make to the process. The key steps of PCAR at the phase of diagnosis are summarized in the following table.

These key steps will be explored in relation to PHLs, communication partners (CPs), and HHPs at the phase of evaluation, diagnosis, and the development of a management plan. Theoretical knowledge and understanding relating to shared

TABLE 8.1 Steps of person-centered audiological rehabilitation at the phase of diagnosis

Evaluation, diagnosis, and identification of individual needs	– Communication
	– Patient needs
	– Clinical significance
Setting of joint rehabilitation goals	– Activity limitation
	– Participation restriction
	– Quality of life
Shared decision making	– Review of the evidence
	– Elicitation of PHL's values and preferences
	– Recommendations and clarification

decision making will enable clinicians to develop and deliver person-centered care (PCC) as a central feature of clinical practice and service provision in audiological rehabilitation.

The process of evaluating hearing loss

The purpose of the evaluation process in relation to hearing loss is to determine the nature, the extent, and the consequences of the loss, in order to implement a remedial intervention that is appropriate and acceptable to the PHLs who are seeking rehabilitative help. The main clinical processes that are involved during the phase of evaluation and diagnosis are: (1) building rapport; (2) understanding the problems experienced by the PHL and their CPs; (3) explaining the results of this evaluation to the PHL and the CPs; and (4) making shared decisions.

As a part of evaluation, audiological assessment is one of the most important steps in the process from diagnostic evaluation to the audiological rehabilitation of the PHL. With the rapid development in technology, as shown in Figure 8.1, there are a range of audiological assessments which provide useful diagnostic information in relation to the nature and degree of hearing loss, on their own as well as when brought together to provide a comprehensive procedural protocol. These measurements contribute to a better understanding of the nature and the degree of hearing loss, together with providing the potential on the underlying pathological auditory mechanisms. Although audiological tests are not discussed in details in this book, some other audiology textbooks are available for such information.

In PCAR, an important aspect of the audiological evaluation concerns how the information it provides might be presented to a PHL, in such a way that his or her understanding of hearing difficulties is enhanced and he or she is provided with information that he or she is able to bring to the decision making he or she shares with the HHP. For example, the results of pure tone audiometry may be contextualized by providing information on the frequency range that is sampled by the procedure, and examples of the kinds of sounds that might be encountered across that frequency range. Combined with this, the range of levels heard by normal listeners,

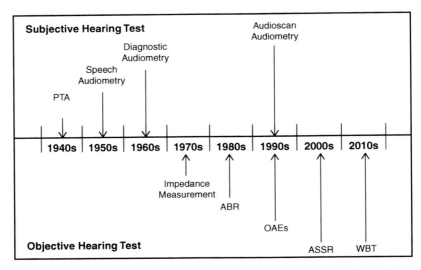

FIGURE 8.1 A range of clinical audiological assessments and their development timeline – subjective and objective hearing tests

together with examples of the levels of typical sounds, may enable the PHL to gain a better understanding of why he or she may be having trouble. The expected effect of the PHL's loss may then be illustrated with reference to the results of speech discrimination testing, and the consequences for this of competing background noise. This information may then be related back to the difficulties that the PHL has described himself/herself experiencing in everyday situations.

With respect to the results of objective hearing tests, the explanation may be most usefully focused on the effect of the alteration to the system being measured. For example, tympanometric results provide information on alterations to the admittance characteristics of the middle ear system. Of importance to the informed decision making of the PHL is the influence of these alterations on hearing and how interventions may help return the middle ear system to "normal" functioning, or compensate for pathological alterations to reduce their effects on activities, participation, and HRQoL related to hearing loss. A similar orientation may be taken to the explanation of otoacoustic emissions (OAEs) and auditory brainstem response (ABR) results, where these can also help to explain some of the limitations imposed by the loss on what may be done to assist the PHL.

While the use of audiometric and physiological measurement procedures is an important aspect of the evaluation of hearing loss, equally important is the inclusion of PHLs' hearing experiences and their perceptions of their own hearing difficulties. The relevance of this was argued in the audiological enablement model proposed by Stephens and Kramer (2009), where normal hearing sensitivity is fundamental for communication, which in turn is important for normal daily life and effective work or study. Therefore, hearing difficulties caused by any kind of auditory disorder will not only hamper effective communication, but will also have emotional and psychological sequelae, and consequently significantly reduce the HRQoL of the PHL.

Drawing on the biopsychosocial model of the WHO-ICF classification (2001), as described in Chapter 2, it is essential to take the evaluation beyond a consideration of aspects of body structure and function to include the effect of the hearing loss on activities and participation, and the influence of personal and environmental factors on these. The importance of this is illustrated by the situation frequently encountered by HHPs: *people with similar types and degrees of hearing loss experience very different types and degrees of hearing-related difficulties.* In part, this may be explained by the variations in the respective activities that make up their daily lives, and the extent of their respective participation in these activities. Consequently the communication situations they encounter will be different, as will their CPs, and they will manage these in different ways.

A number of questionnaire instruments have been used to assess the situations or difficulties experienced by people with hearing loss. One such example is the Hearing Handicap Questionnaire (HHQ; Gatehouse and Noble, 2004). Although measures such as these have useful sections on the PHL's "emotional" and "social" aspects related to hearing loss, there is generally a limited emphasis on the psychosocial effects of hearing loss. Moreover, these structured types of questionnaires tend to approach the PHL's difficulties from the standpoint of the HHPs rather than that of the PHL.

An evaluation instrument employing open-ended questions offers an alternative approach to the assessment of the difficulties experienced by the PHL. These permit the eliciting of difficulties as they are experienced by the PHL, rather than constraining the PHLs' responses to the items included in a structured questionnaire, which may or may not be relevant to their needs. Open-ended questions offer a useful and relevant tool for highlighting the specific concerns of PHLs. For these to be effective, though, it is essential that they include a consideration of the difficulties in relation to the hearing loss that the PHL experiences across a number of key areas (Table 8.2).

The role of hearing healthcare professionals

According to the evaluation and diagnostic nature in hearing healthcare, various studies have suggested that HHPs play an important role in many ways as listed below:

- taking a case history;
- conducting audiological assessments;
- providing essential feedback to PHLs on the basis of information obtained from the evaluation process (e.g., audiological testing results, subjective patient evaluation of experience and perceptions);
- debriefing the PHL about his or her symptoms and assessment results;
- providing suggestions on possible intervention options; and consequent management and prognosis.

To achieve these by playing such a role safely and professionally, hearing health professionals must gain essential competence and experience in the field of audiology and related areas. Such competence is expected by audiology professional bodies, and

TABLE 8.2 Summary of key areas of difficulty arising from hearing loss

Category	Key areas of difficulties
"Live" speech	• General conversation • Group conversation • Speech in noise • Meetings • TV and radio
Sound	• Warning devices (e.g., doorbell, phone ringing, fire alarm) • Music • Localization
Social aspects	• Employment difficulties • Difficulty interacting with strangers • Difficulties with participation in social situations • Isolation
Psychological aspects	• Becoming irritable, nervous, or moody • Loneliness • Embarrassment • Ignorance • Feelings of being undermined • Feelings of being a strain on family • Depression

may be completed through accredited educational courses and work-based learning. Education and experience should include coverage of fundamental components, including subject-specific knowledge, clinical skills, capability in terms of logical reasoning and problem-solving, and quick judgment of which approach to use and when, and the ability to evaluate and use evidence from research (Epstein and Hundert, 2002). As shown in Table 8.3, HHPs are required to master and use knowledge to solve real-life problems, together with integrating biomedical and psychosocial data in clinics.

Furthermore, with increasing clinical practice and accumulating clinical experience, HHPs would have a better understanding of insight knowledge and clinical skills in terms of dealing appropriately with more difficult management problems, and consequently provide high quality hearing healthcare for PHLs. In the meantime, it is essential to reflect on daily practice, which allows practitioners to further develop their professional skills, and therefore improve quality of care, which is beneficial for the individuals and the communities being served (Epstein and Hundert, 2002).

Interpretation of clinical significance by hearing healthcare professionals

The concept of clinical significance refers to the value or importance that is attached by the PHL to the effect of functional changes, in terms of whether or

TABLE 8.3 Main domains of professional competence in audiology (adopted from Epstein and Hundert, 2002)

Theoretical knowledge and integrative skills

- Core knowledge in audiology and related areas
- Applying knowledge to real-world situations
- Abstract problem solving
- Self-directed acquisition of new knowledge
- Recognizing gaps in knowledge
- Generating questions
- Reviewing the evidence
- Using resources (e.g., published evidence, colleagues)
- Information management

Clinical skills

- Various ranges of audiological assessments and intervention
- Linking basic and clinical knowledge across disciplines
- Learning from experience
- Reflective practice
- Managing uncertainty

Communication and relationships

- Basic communication skills
- Engagement
- Team work
- Handling conflict

Affective/moral and habits of mind

- Commitment
- Caring and respect for patients
- Responsiveness to patients and society
- Attentiveness

not the functional change has a meaningful effect on the everyday life of the PHL or other people with whom the PHL interacts (Kazdin, 1999). Evaluating clinical significance in terms of the effect of hearing loss on the functioning of the PHL is a critical dimension of interpretation. Importantly, the information provided by the PHL provides a context for the audiometric and physiological measures that support this aspect of the evaluation and diagnostic process. Moreover, the interpretation of clinical significance represents an important phase in terms of the decision making and management strategy, including possible intervention approaches, as well as extending to prevention, education, and rehabilitation (Kazdin, 1999).

When the audiologist refers to change as clinically significant, it needs to reflect consideration of the question "What does the change mean in real-life situations for the person with hearing loss?" Thus while a change in hearing may have occurred, its significance for the PHL may range from minimal to considerable, depending on the effects of the change on the PHL's daily activities (activity limitation), and also the extent to which the activity limitation restricts his or her participation in social interactions. Participation restrictions may be associated with a number of social and economic difficulties such as social isolation, social and economic deprivation, and the inability to participate in the labor market (Royal National Institute for the Deaf, 2006).

By contrast, a hearing loss may not have a significant effect for some PHLs, due to their lifestyles. An example of this may be an elderly person living alone at home. Therefore, the interpretation of whether or not a change of hearing status should be interpreted as having clinical significance needs to take into consideration psychosocial information, as well as the judgments of significance made by PHLs themselves. The appropriate interpretation of clinical significance constitutes a core dimension of PCAR.

The communication experience of persons with hearing loss and their communication partners

All PHLs need to be provided with clear information, particularly in the light of its importance for enabling PHLs to contribute to the determination of the clinical significance of a hearing loss. However, the communication exchange between HHPs and PHLs is not always as effective and efficient as it should be because of a number of influencing factors. These include deaf awareness and audiological knowledge, communication mode, and the severity of the hearing loss. For example, PHLs may have trouble with oral modes of communication when their hearing loss is severe or profound. A Royal National Institute for the Deaf project report (2006) assessed PHLs' experiences of communication using a "Health Care Satisfaction Questionnaire for Deaf and Hard of Hearing People." In the multiple stepwise regression analysis, PHLs with severe or profound hearing loss were more likely to report poorer communication in the domain of general clarity, and particularly in the technical explanatory domains of clinician-PHL dialogue (Royal National Institute for the Deaf, 2006). Moreover, another study was carried out to investigate the effect of language barriers on PHLs when health professionals used medical jargon (Iezzoni et al., 2004). The results showed that medical staff did not fully recognize the implications of the communication barriers experienced by PHLs, and consequently they had fundamental misconceptions about effective communication modalities, which are findings confirmed by others. In particular, clinicians often believe that note writing and lip reading provide a basis for effective communication. However, only 30–45 percent of English sounds are unambiguously visible on lips, and note writing often fails as well (McEwan and Anton-Culver, 1988).

Although PHLs are satisfied with their healthcare in general, because of the nature of their disablement, the barriers and difficulties they encounter are most prevalent in the communication domain. The greatest difficulty and dissatisfaction as they describe relates to listening to *live speech*. Examples of this are difficulties "in hearing name called in the waiting room," "in hearing nurses or doctors or receptionists," and "on the phone when making appointment" (Royal National Institute for the Deaf, 2006). The other main problems listed under the category of communication difficulties were deaf awareness on the part of health professionals, which related to their understanding of, and sensitivity to, the needs of PHLs, and an understanding on the part of health professionals of psychological effects of hearing loss on PHLs. These results suggest that special attention regarding these aspects needs to be given to PHLs. This will permit HHPs to contribute to the adaptation of the communication encounter with PHLs in ways that will help to address the barriers and difficulties experienced by PHLs, providing a basis of communication that will permit safe, timely, efficient PCC.

Effective communication is one of the most important components of the phase of evaluation and diagnosis for the PHL (Grenness et al., 2014a, 2014b; Grenness et al., 2015). From PHLs' perspective, being provided with better knowledge about the hearing loss and its implications is likely to help them to describe more clearly their experience of the change to their hearing. Effective communication will also contribute to PHLs' understanding of the significance of the interpretations placed by the HHP on the data collected during the evaluation, consequently permitting them to benefit more from intervention and rehabilitation. In order to provide a basis for effective communication, HHPs should try to establish the PHL's perception of the problem, check the PHL's knowledge and understanding of hearing loss, and respond appropriately to the PHL's feelings about the evaluation and diagnostic process. In support, there are a number of aspects of communication to which the

TABLE 8.4 Summary of aspects of communication

Aspects of communication relating to the HHP

- Language level (word choice, phrase length, grammatical complexity)
- Prosody, accent, dialect
- Speed of speech, speed of information transmission
- Nonverbal communication (facial expression and eye contact, gesture to facilitate communication, body language, space and proximity)
- Conveying affect, typically neutral to positive (attention and listening, understanding and empathy, authenticity and congruence, openness)

Aspects of communication relating to the HHP's responses to the PHL

- Responding to aspects of the PHL's speech intelligibility (checking and interpreting, facilitating and cueing, compensating and circumlocution)
- Responding to aspects of the PHL's language (simplifying, recasting, providing alternative symbols or medium of communication)
- Responding to aspects of PHL's understanding (orienting and making explicit the implicit, simplifying and reconfiguring, contextualizing and cueing, explaining and providing additional or alternative information, developing a sense of the PHL's frame of reference and offering alternative points of view, discerning what may be unstated

HHP might give attention. These are summarized in Table 8.4, and include aspects of the HHP's communication and the ways in which the HHP may respond to, and facilitate, the communication of the PHL.

In addition to the interaction of the HHP with the PHL, it is important to consider the contribution that the CP of the PHL is able to make to effective communication during the phase of evaluation and diagnosis. The CP plays a valuable role in terms of providing support to the person with hearing loss, particularly at the entry point to the hearing healthcare system. The CP may know the PHL well in terms of his or her personality, educational background, health history, language background (primary language and additional language), and cultural background, and therefore they can bring a unique combination of experience and intellectual capital to the communication challenges in the evaluation phase. In cases where normal communication may be negatively affected by the hearing loss, the involvement of a CP can make a valuable contribution to the communication process and the evaluation of the effect of the hearing loss on activities and participation. Iezzoni and colleagues (2004) have suggested that CPs may be able to provide useful information about a PHL's communication style, preferences for interaction with individuals or groups, extent of daily use of reading and writing, sense of humor, and sophistication of vocabulary and language usage. In addition, the involvement of CPs can also help to develop a diverse range of communication strategies by addressing communication difficulties, and therefore improve communication processes (Grenness et al., 2015). However, an important consideration for the involvement of CPs during the evaluation phase is to ensure that they, the PHL, and the HHP are all equal partners in promoting effective communication, and that the primary role of the PHL in the evaluation phase is not undermined.

Shared decision making

In the 1970s, George Engel challenged the biomedical model of healthcare, and he formulated a biopsychosocial diagnosis and treatment model (Engel, 1977) that endeavored to address the psychological and social aspects of medicine. Since then, the PCC has become increasingly popular. This approach suggests that persons with health difficulties should be encouraged to be active participants in their healthcare through the creation of a power-balanced therapeutic relationship with the healthcare professional (Grenness et al., 2014a). Because of its positive effect on health outcomes, PCC has been widely welcomed by people who experience chronic health difficulties. According to the ICF, a key component of PCC is to involve persons with health difficulties in the healthcare process, particularly in the process of diagnosis and intervention. Involving people in their healthcare decisions is internationally increasingly recognized as important for matching their care with their preferences, and for improving the safety and quality of that care.

In PCC, clinicians are encouraged to explore how people perceive their symptoms, what they believe is causing their health difficulties, and how these affect their daily functioning (Dolan, 2008). PCC contributes to greater satisfaction with, and adherence to, treatment, increased willingness to self-manage, improvement in health status, and reduction in symptoms. An important feature of PCC is shared decision making. In Whitney and colleagues' 2004 study, shared decision making was defined as "a collaborative endeavour in which patient and physician share not only information and intuitions but also the making of decisions." It is a process in which HHPs and PHLs work together to clarify treatment, management, or self-management support goals, and share information about options and preferred outcomes with the aim of reaching mutual agreement on the best course of action. Shared decision making enables PHLs and their CPs to arrive at agreed decisions by bringing together PHLs' understandings and preferences, scientific evidence on outcomes, and HHPs' expertise in the integration of evidence and individual clinical circumstances and values.

Several studies have identified factors that might affect patient preferences for involvement in the process of shared decision making. For example, a review paper by Say and colleagues (2006) highlighted factors such as PHLs' experience of illness and medical care, the diagnosis and their health status, the type of decision the PHLs need to make, the amount of knowledge they have acquired about their condition, and the interactions and relationships they experience with health professionals. It is important for HHPs to consider these factors and develop sensitive ways of empowering PHLs so that they may experience the benefits associated with their involvement in the process of decision making.

The key steps of a shared decision-making process during audiological diagnosis and evaluation are shown as follows:

1. *Set goals and intervention options:* Once the evaluation has been completed and the findings have been integrated, initial goal setting may be explored in the light of the available options. The PHL is then asked to prioritize these goals in terms of the possible effects they may have on her or his life, and to discuss with the HHP how such goals should be approached.

2. *Review the evidence to identify the optimal option(s):* This step of the process requires that the HHP critically assesses the evidence, and identifies how well the optimal option is likely to meet the goal, through comparing and integrating all of the information obtained from the evaluation.

3. *Elicit PHL's values and preferences:* In this step the HHP needs to respect the PHL's right to choose their preferred hearing care and audiological intervention. In doing so, they may need to strike a balance between their own professional views and the preferences of the PHL in order to arrive at a mutually agreed decision.

4. *Offer recommendations:* The purpose of this step is to ensure that PHLs are fully informed about the options they have selected. This involves providing them with reliable evidence-based information on the likely benefits and harm of interventions or actions, including the feasibility of these and any uncertainties

and risks, relating these back to their preferences, and practical considerations relating to the implementation of these options.

5.   *Check for clarity and understanding:* For decision making to be shared equally between the PHL, HHP, and CP, it is important that the basis for the decisions taken rests on a common understanding. The role of the HHP during this step is to ensure that a common understanding exists and, when this is not the case, to implement strategies outlined in Table 8.3 in order to address the difficulty.

6.   *Make a shared decision:* The role of the HHP during this step is to clearly state the decision that has been reached, supported by the information, evidence, values, and preferences that have been discussed as a part of the process of evaluation and diagnosis. In doing so the HHP will summarize by:

   a.   providing clear reliable information supported by evidence;
   b.   outlining intervention, care and support options, and possible outcomes and risks;
   c.   examining and discussing options and preferences; and
   d.   communicating how the PHL's preferences will be implemented.

Summary

With the development of scientific and technological advances, audiological assessments provide sensitive, accurate, and reliable information on not only the nature of hearing loss, but also some of the mechanisms behind these. However, sophisticated information may confuse PHLs if it is not interpreted meaningfully by clinicians. Alongside technical developments, there has been a shift in the type of information that is considered important in audiological evaluation and diagnosis. Changes have also occurred in the allocation of responsibility for determining the relative importance of information and decisions made based on it. This has placed a demand on the HHP to develop new models of understanding the PHL's experience of hearing loss, and new models of clinical interaction with PHLs in order to give effect to PCAR. Patient-centered communication and shared decision making are relatively new concepts that are yet to be fully integrated into the organizational culture of hearing healthcare settings.

References

Dolan, J., 2008. Shared decision-making – transferring research into practice: the Analytic Hierarchy Process (AHP). *Patient Education and Counseling*, 73(3), pp. 418–425.

Engel, G., 1977. The need for a new medical model: a challenge for biomedicine. *Science*, 196, pp. 129–136.

Epstein, R. and Hundert, E., 2002. Defining and assessing professional competence. *Journal of the American Medical Association*, 287(2), pp. 226–235.

Gagné, J., Jennings, M., and Southall, K., 2009. The international classification of functioning: implications and applications to audiological rehabilitation. In J. J. Montano and J. B. Spitzer (Eds.), *Adult audiologic rehabilitation*, 2nd ed., pp. 517–534. San Diego, CA: Plural Publishing, Inc.

Gatehouse, S. and Noble, W., 2004. The speech, spatial, and qualities of hearing scale (SSQ). *International Journal of Audiology*, 43, pp. 85–99.

Grenness, C., Hickson, L., Laplante-Lévesque, A., and Davidson, B., 2014a. Patient-centred audiological rehabilitation: perspectives of older adults who own hearing aids. *International Journal of Audiology*, 53(S1), pp. 68S–75S.

Grenness, C., Hickson, L., Laplante-Lévesque, A., and Davidson, B., 2014b. Patient-centred care: a review for rehabilitative audiologists. *International Journal of Audiologists*, 53(S1), pp. 60S–67S.

Grenness, C., Hickson, L., Laplante-Lévesque, A., Meyer, C., and Davidson, B., 2015. Communication patterns in audiologic rehabilitation history-taking: audiologists, patients, and their companions. *Ear and Hearing*, 36(2), pp. 191–204.

Iezzoni, L., O'day, B., Killeen, M., and Harker, H., 2004. Communicating about health care: observations from persons who are deaf or hard of hearing. *Annals of Internal Medicine*, 140, pp. 356–362.

Kazdin, A., 1999. The meanings and measurement of clinical significance. *Journal of Consulting and Clinical Psychology*, 67(3), pp. 332–339.

McEwan, E. and Anton-Culver, H., 1988. The medical communication of deaf patients. *Journal of Family Practice*, 26, pp. 289–291.

Royal National Institute for the Deaf, 2006. *Satisfaction with quality of health care for deaf and hard of hearing people in Wales*. Swansea University, Wales, UK: Royal National Institute for the Deaf.

Say, R., Murtagh, M., and Thomson, R., 2006. Patients' preference for involvement in medical decision-making: a narrative review. *Patient Education and Counseling*, 60(2), pp. 102–114.

Stephens, D. and Kramer, S., 2009. *Living with hearing difficulties: the process of enablement*. Chichester, West Sussex, UK: John Wiley & Sons, Ltd.

Whitney, S., McGuirem, A., and McCullough, L., 2004. A typology of shared decision making, informed consent, and simple consent. *Annals of Internal Medicine*, 140, pp. 54–59.

World Health Organization, 2001. *International Classification of Functioning, Disability and Health (ICF)*. Geneva, Switzerland: World Health Organization.

9

REHABILITATION

Learning and adapting to new methods

Vinay Swarnalatha Nagaraj

Introduction

In this chapter, the "rehabilitation" phase of the journey is discussed. This phase demonstrates real commitment from the person with hearing loss (PHL) to remove and/or reduce limitations and to improve functioning. As the hearing loss is chronic in nature in most cases, the PHL will experience this phase several times in their life course. The outcome of this process lays the foundation for success or failure in an attempt to resolve their hearing loss.

The rehabilitation of the individual with a hearing loss depends largely upon the extent and the type of hearing loss. Increased hearing thresholds leading to the inaudibility of speech is a major contributing factor for poor understanding of speech. However, for PHL with greater severity of loss, providing equivalent speech information at high levels to both normal hearing and hearing impaired persons often results in poorer speech understanding for the impaired persons (Ching et al., 1998; Hogan and Turner, 1998). For a majority of individuals with a conductive hearing loss (i.e., problem in external and middle ear), prescription of medications or surgery might be recommended. On the other hand, individuals with a sensorineural hearing loss (i.e., problem in inner ear or beyond in the auditory system) require intervention in the form of hearing aid fitting. Despite its high prevalence and consequences for health outcomes, hearing loss is largely underdiagnosed and thus undertreated. Studies also report that, in certain cases, providing audibility actually reduces the speech recognition abilities in persons with sensorineural hearing loss. This might be one of the reasons that people who have a hearing loss are reluctant to seek further help.

Consequences of hearing loss

The function of the auditory system is significant in day-to-day activities of home, work, social, and other situations. The process of auditory recognition is a means of communication of the spoken language. Previous studies have highlighted psychological implications of hearing loss, which may include everything from embarrassment, shame, guilt, and anger. See Chapter 1 for more details about the consequences of hearing loss.

Process from awareness to rehabilitation uptake

Some of the studies have reported the process involved in patients understanding the problems of hearing loss and following-up with help seeking and rehabilitation (Mahoney et al., 1996). It is observed that many factors co-exist that affect the outcome of hearing loss rehabilitation. In general, it is observed that the process between being aware of having a hearing loss and acceptance of requiring rehabilitation can be a long one. Identifying and accepting oneself the existence of a hearing loss is an important step towards effective rehabilitation. In the study by Mahoney and colleagues (1996), 95 patients were observed in two audiology centers (London and Cardiff), and were questioned as to the primary person who motivated them to first seek help for their hearing loss. The results indicated that only a minority of patients reported that they were self-motivated and that in the majority, especially with the older patients and those not working outside the home, it was a family member who persuaded the patient to consult his doctor (Mahoney et al., 1996). In a study by Carson (2005), it was reported that older women moved away from seeking quality help for hearing loss assessment and rehabilitation. Sometimes the hearing problem might not be noticeable to the patient themselves but may be noticed by significant others. A typical instance of such a situation can be:

> I had not thought that I have a hearing loss until my wife mentioned to me that I set the TV volume high and I sometimes do not respond to her while she talks to me from the kitchen.
>
> *(70 year old, male, India)*

This leads us to think what factors then might prompt an individual with a hearing loss to seek help. A study by Meyer and Hickson (2012) indicated that individuals are more likely to seek help for hearing loss and/or uptake rehabilitation options if they have a significant hearing loss (e.g., moderate degree or greater) and/or self-report hearing disability (e.g., activity limitations and participation restrictions). The study also observed that older individuals are more likely to seek help if they perceive their hearing ability as poor. In certain cases, the advantages obtained from wearing a hearing aid to improve communication abilities outweigh the disadvantages of living with a hearing loss without seeking help. Often significant members of the family need to be involved to have increased support for hearing assessment and rehabilitation of the patient with hearing loss. Hence, these factors promote the patients to seek help for hearing rehabilitation through the use of hearing aids.

Previous literature has addressed the process involved in the patient journey for assessment and rehabilitation of hearing loss (Grutters et al., 2007). For example, Grutters and colleagues (2007) evaluated the attitudes of professionals (General Practitioners [GPs], hearing aid dispensers, otolaryngologists [ear, nose, and throat specialists], and clinical audiologists) and patients towards a direct referral pathway for hearing aid fitting (dispenser) as opposed to an alternative route (via the GP and ENT specialist and clinical audiologist). The PHL, the GPs, and the hearing aid dispensers generally had positive attitudes towards the direct pathway, whereas the ENT doctors and the clinical audiologists had negative concerns about the direct referral.

Stephens and Kramer (2009) suggest that the patient with hearing loss can be broadly categorized into four groups based on their rehabilitation types, which include: (1) Positively motivated without complicating factors; (2) Positively motivated with complicating factors; (3) Want help, but reject a key component; and (4) Deny any problems.

Individuals usually with a mild hearing loss might not accept that they have a hearing loss. Some of the experiences can be as follows:

> I do not have a hearing problem unless people speak to me softly.
> *(65 year old male, India, has not sought help for hearing rehabilitation)*

> I do not have a hearing loss, but I can get a hearing evaluation done. In all probabilities I do not need a hearing aid.
> *(67 year old female, India, after suggestions from family members that she needs to get her hearing checked)*

It often happens that the individual is not willing to accept that he/she has a hearing loss and if they do agree to a hearing evaluation, motivation towards obtaining a hearing aid is poor. Knudsen and colleagues (2010) have described the stages involved in patient help seeking for rehabilitation. The main body of literature divides the patient journey into three stages: 1) the stage prior to help seeking and uptake of hearing aids; 2) the period covering the process of the fitting; and 3) the short- or long-term period after the hearing aid fitting (Knudsen et al., 2010). There have been studies that have investigated the factors that contribute to a patient's decision in actively seeking help in terms of assessment of their hearing and/or in terms of rehabilitation. Knudsen et al. (2010) studied the factors of help seeking, uptake, use, and satisfaction in different stages of patients' hearing assessment and rehabilitation journeys.

Hearing aid acceptance has been widely discussed recently as being necessary for the success of hearing rehabilitation. Studies indicate that the whole process of help-seeking and acceptance may take a long duration and one must understand the importance of motivation and awareness regarding different stages in this process. See Chapter 6 for more details regarding the acceptance of the rehabilitation process.

Rehabilitation options

The role of the audiologist in providing an effective counseling and communication strategy-oriented aural rehabilitation program is important. This is because despite the large prevalence of hearing loss, the motivation of the patients to wear hearing aids is still in its infancy. A relatively small proportion of adults with hearing loss seek help for their hearing problems and use hearing aids. In addition, it is also observed that not all patients who are provided with hearing aids use them, wear them, or are satisfied with them (Lupsakko et al., 2005). These descriptions can be well supported by patient experiences as observed above.

At the outset, it is important to discuss the rehabilitation options for PHLs. A patient with a hearing loss has a variety of options for rehabilitation. The options for rehabilitation can be depicted in the form of a diagram as shown in Figure 9.1.

Once the patient is motivated and understands the need for rehabilitation, it might be worth being aware of the importance of the rehabilitation options. Successful communication requires the efforts of all people significantly involved in a conversation with the patient with hearing loss. Even when the PHL wears hearing aids and active listening devices, it is crucial that communication partners (CPs) involved in the communication process with the patient understand the process involved in using effective strategies.

As shown in the figure, the rehabilitation options can be classified based on the techniques utilized for communication:

• use of communication strategies;
• use of technological options; and
• a combination of communication strategies and technological options.

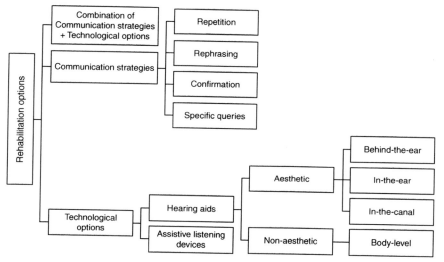

FIGURE 9.1 Rehabilitation options for adults with hearing loss

Use of communication strategies

This section presents a brief discussion about communication strategies. However, see Chapter 11 for an in-depth discussion about communication and conversation.

Repetition

It might be highlighted that the use of repetition or request to present the stimuli again improves understanding between conversational partners (Tye-Murray, 1991).
Example:

Person 1: Did you know that Tom has been appointed as the new manager for the company?
Patient: I am sorry, what did you say?
Person 1: Did you know that Tom has been appointed as the new manager for the company?

In this strategy, the patient uses an open-ended question, not specifically targeting the parts of the information that he/she could not hear. This situation might occur if the PHL was not attending to the stimuli or in an unfavorable environmental condition such as high background noise as in a cocktail party effect.

Rephrasing

This strategy is effective in communication. The use of repair strategies or request for clarification for rephrasing is also shown to be effective (Tye-Murray, 1991).
Example:

Person 1: Did you know that Tom has been appointed as the new manager for the company?
Patient: Sorry, what?
Person 1: Tom is the new manager for Alpha Company.

A rearrangement of the stimuli might result in better understanding of the content. This will result in rephrasing and a part of the stimulus is repeated for effective communication.

Confirmation

This strategy involves the PHL requesting for clarification for specific or overall information. Requests for specific clarification are viewed more favorably by the speaker than non-specific requests (Caissie and Gibson, 1997).

Example:

Person 1: Did you know that Tom has been appointed as the new manager for the company?
Patient: Is Tom appointed as the new manager for the company?
Person 1: Yes, you are right.

Specific queries

This strategy is a modification of the repetition strategy where the patient directs his question to specific content. Here, in this strategy, the PHL does not use an open-ended question. The questions indicate answers requiring who, what, where, or how. Tactfully ask the PHL if they understood you, or ask leading questions so you know your message got across.

Example:

Person 1: Did you know that Tom has been appointed as the new manager for the company?
Patient: Who is appointed as the new manager for the company?
Person 1: Tom.

Technological options

Generally, the technological options include (1) hearing aids and/or (2) assistive listening devices.

The goal of this chapter is to highlight the effective forms of rehabilitation for a PHL. This topic will not be described in detail as the scope of this book is concentrated more on highlighting overall rehabilitation options rather than offering information about technological tools for rehabilitation. A major difficulty of listeners with hearing loss in understanding speech arises from the loss of audibility of some parts of the speech signal that are important for recognition. Therefore, hearing aid amplification systems often aim to restore audibility of those portions of the speech spectrum that are below the listeners' thresholds. It is generally assumed that speech recognition will be optimized when audibility is maximized. However, research on the effect of audibility on speech recognition scores has demonstrated that audibility alone cannot adequately predict the reduced speech recognition of PHLs with moderate or severe losses (Dubno et al., 1989; Vinay and Moore, 2007). This suggests that compensating for the loss of audibility may not always be helpful in individuals with hearing loss. This factor leads us to discuss the next section related to a combination of communication strategies and technological options.

Combination of communication strategies and technological options

A combination of communication strategies and technological options has been shown to be an effective means of transferring information in a conversation with a PHL. Many factors are useful in providing effective communication for these individuals. It is important that the person in conversation faces the PHL on the same level whenever possible. It has been shown that a PHL can derive useful information from the speaker such as lip reading cues, emotions, and other important factors. It is also important that the speaker faces in a certain direction so that the light shines on his/her face.

If the speaker's face is adequately visible in bright light conditions, this might help the PHL get important cues of articulation and emotion related to the topic.

It is always advised that the speaker avoid speaking from a distance or from another room. Not being able to see each other when carrying out a conversation results in difficulty understanding what was actually said in the conversation for a PHL.

> My wife speaks to me from the kitchen. I find it hard to listen to her most of the time since her voice is feeble and I do not get the context of the conversation.
>
> *(Male, 65 years old)*

Quite often, the speaker is unaware of the rate of speech while conversing with a PHL. The speaker naturally tends to speak at his/her "normal" conversation rate; however, the PHL might find it difficult to understand and process the stimuli. Hence it is advised that the speaker talks clearly, slowly, and articulates every sound as much as possible, but speaks naturally to result in effective communication. Shouting distorts the sound of speech and may make speech reading more difficult.

Another important feature that must be understood is that the speaker needs to provide his/her introduction before starting a conversation. This helps in two ways for a PHL – first, the patient finds adequate time to prepare to understand the actual conversation, and second, the patient acquires important information about the details of the speaker and the context of the conversation. This gives the listener a chance to focus attention and reduces the chance of missing words at the beginning of the conversation. Quite often, it happens to a person conversing in a foreign language in the learning stage. A native speaker of that language frequently changes the context of the conversation, and then the learner of the foreign language often finds it difficult to understand the conversation due to topic "jumps."

Example for conversation "jumps":

Native speaker: Hi how is it going?
Language learner: It is going fine here and how are you?
Native speaker: The "Rosenborg" football team won the match yesterday. Did you watch the match?

Example for model conversation:

> *Person 1:* Hi, my name is Jim and I work in Alpha Company. How about you?
> *Patient:* Nice to meet you Jim, my name is Tom and I am your colleague.
> *Person 1:* It is nice that you work in the same company as mine, when did you join here?
> *Patient:* I joined yesterday.

It is important that the speaker avoids a rapid rate of speech and should avoid using sentences that are too complex. Recognize that everyone, especially the hard-of-hearing, has a harder time hearing and understanding when ill or tired. A simple sentence would serve a long way in the understanding of speech for the patient with hearing loss. If you are eating, chewing, smoking, etc. while talking, it is important to know that a person with normal hearing would find it difficult to understand the speech. Also, hand movements in front of the face can interfere with the ability of the PHL to speech read.

> *Person 1:* Hi, my name is Jim and I am your neighbor. May I borrow your snow shovel for today, since we did not manage to buy one yesterday?

The above example depicts the complexity of the sentence and information bombardment to the patient with a hearing loss. A puzzled look may indicate misunderstanding. Take turns speaking and avoid interrupting other speakers. A better conversation model would be:

> *Person 1:* Hi, my name is Jim.
> *Patient:* Hi, I am Tom.
> *Person 1:* Can I borrow your snow shovel?
> *Patient:* Yes, you can.
> *Person 1:* I am sorry to ask you this, but we forgot to buy one.
> *Patient:* That's fine.

If the PHL hears better in one ear than the other or in other words, the patient has a unilateral hearing loss, the speaker should try to position himself/herself towards the better ear. Also, one should be aware of possible distortion of sounds for the PHL. Usually, a PHL perceives distortion in the speech stimuli due to altered ear mechanisms. They may hear your voice, but still may have difficulty understanding some words. One of the biggest complaints of the PHL is difficulty understanding speech when there is background noise. The speaker should try to minimize extraneous noise when talking. Some PHLs are very sensitive to loud sounds. This reduced tolerance for loud sounds is not uncommon. Avoid situations where there will be loud sounds when possible. If the PHL has difficulty understanding a particular phrase or word, try to find a different way of saying the same thing, rather than repeating the original words over and over. This helps the PHL to understand the spoken message better. As much as possible the PHL must be acquainted with the general topic of the conversation. If the topic of discussion changes drastically, then inform the patient what you are talking about beforehand. In a group setting, it is important to repeat questions or important information before continuing with the actual conversation. If you are giving specific information – such as time, place, or phone numbers – to someone who is experiencing hearing loss, then it would be ideal to have the information repeated by the person experiencing hearing loss just to know if the transfer of information has been complete. In terms of phonetics of speech sounds, many numbers/words/speech can sound alike. Whenever possible, provide additional and useful information in writing. One of the best approaches would be to enroll in aural rehabilitation classes with the PHL to learn techniques and strategies for effective communication.

Effect of personal and environmental factors on rehabilitation success and the role of ICF and Universal Design in hearing rehabilitation

A diminished ability to hear and communicate is frustrating, and influences the affected individuals as well as other people in their environment. The concept of universal design for hearing focuses on the design and composition of an environment that can be accessed and used by most people, including those with and without hearing loss, to the greatest possible extent. The design of an environment that is flexible and meets the needs of a wide range of users can eliminate or minimize communication difficulties for a PHL and to CPs in the family. As discussed earlier in the chapter, present-day strategies for rehabilitation often include providing adaptive devices to PHLs that are targeted primarily at the person. However, equally important is the role of communication strategies for the patient. The family members also often experience the communication difficulties experienced by the PHL. Many studies have concluded that family members are significantly affected by the PHL's condition and may often initiate the need for the PHL's audiological rehabilitation (Hétu et al., 1993). The concept of Universal Design, however, includes all individuals, with and without hearing loss, associated with effective communication. Family members are significantly affected by the consequences of hearing loss and can potentially play an important role in a client's hearing rehabilitation. In accordance with the concepts of Universal Design, the World Health Organization's (WHO) International Classification of Functioning, Disability and Health (ICF) classifies the effect of hearing loss on significant others as a "*third-party disability.*" The significant others are considered as those individuals who play an important role in the everyday life of the PHL. Rehabilitation professionals often need to involve significant others in the rehabilitation of the PHL (see Chapter 4). PHL understanding of the rehabilitation options such as hearing aid and assistive listening devices and shared decision making are important. The involvement of the significant others helps to shift the rehabilitation focus from person-centered to family-centered care in accordance with the principles of Universal Design for hearing.

Care and maintenance of a hearing aid

Cleaning a hearing aid is a service generally provided by a hearing healthcare professional/audiologist every time you visit the clinic, but having knowledge about the care and maintenance will serve as a good practice to follow at home. For an effective rehabilitation program in the journey of a PHL, understanding the importance of care and maintenance of a hearing aid is essential. This information will help prevent the need for repair and will prolong the life of the hearing aid. Thereby, the PHL obtains immense satisfaction and can avail full benefits of a hearing aid while in use. An audiologist needs to highlight this information during the counseling of the PHL. The audiologist must inform the patient about simple techniques that might be useful in repairing and maintaining the working of the hearing aid. Aspects such as awareness of the different parts of the hearing aid and its functions should be communicated. In addition to keeping the hearing device in good condition, routinely checking the hearing aid enables the wearer to ensure there are no visible damages or issues. Monitoring the life of the batteries according to the number of hours used is important. Simple techniques like replacing batteries, checking the acoustic tube for moisture and blockage, and avoiding feedback sound should be highlighted. In addition, care should be taken for the hearing aids to be switched off before going to sleep to avoid unnecessary wastage of batteries. Hearing aid acoustic tubes and sound entrance are prone to build up, which thus cause blockage to these tubes. Hence, the PHL needs to be aware of cleaning the hearing aids to remove the blockage. Hearing aids should be professionally cleaned once or twice a year, or more often if required. Hearing care practitioners have specialized instruments they use to clean hearing aids, without causing damage to your hearing aids, as well as adequate training and experience. If the PHL finds it difficult to solve the issues that the hearing aid device has, then it is best to consult the hearing care professional to check the device.

Summary

Based on the experiences presented in this chapter, it is important that the PHL realizes the importance of hearing assessment and, if needed, about rehabilitation. Experiences and studies have indicated that significant others play an important role in the rehabilitation of the PHL. It is important to realize that the patient journey includes a team approach consisting of the PHL, family members/care-givers, and/ or significant others with whom the patient sustains daily communication abilities. As described in this chapter, the rehabilitation options for the PHL vary according to the extent and the type of hearing loss. One must remember the importance of understanding and treating the symptoms rather than basing the rehabilitation options on the diagnosis itself. CPs play an important role in providing motivation and guidance for help seeking for a PHL.

The role of environmental factors should be taken into consideration during the rehabilitation of the PHL. Basic knowledge about hearing aid function and maintenance will go a long way in terms of success in hearing rehabilitation for a person with a hearing loss. Audiologists, patients, and family members need to work in co-ordination to produce the best outcome in such instances.

References

Caissie, R. and Gibson, C., 1997. The effectiveness of repair strategies used by people with hearing losses and their conversational partners. *Volta Review*, 99(4), pp. 203–218.

Carson, A., 2005. "What brings you here today?" The role of self-assessment in help-seeking for age-related hearing loss. *Journal of Aging Studies*, 19(2), pp. 185–200.

Ching, T.Y.C., Dillon, H., and Byrne, D., 1998. Speech recognition of hearing-impaired listeners: predictions from audibility and the limited role of high-frequency amplification. *Journal of the Acoustical Society of America*, 103, pp. 1128–1140.

Dubno, J., Dirks, D., and Schaefer, A., 1989. Stop-consonant recognition for normal-hearing listeners and listeners with high-frequency hearing loss. II: Articulation index predictions. *Journal of the Acoustical Society of America*, 85(1), pp. 355–364.

Grutters, J., Horst, F., Joore, M., Verschuure, H., Dreschler, W., and Anteunis, L., 2007. Potential barriers and facilitators for implementation of an integrated care pathway for hearing-impaired persons: an exploratory survey among patients and professionals. *BMC Health Services Research*, 7(1), p. 1.

Hétu, R., Jones, L., and Getty, L., 1993. The impact of acquired hearing impairment on intimate relationships: implications for rehabilitation. *Audiology*, 32, pp. 363–381.

Hogan, C. and Turner, C., 1998. High frequency audibility: benefits for hearing-impaired listeners. *Journal of the Acoustical Society of America*, 104, pp. 432–441.

Knudsen, L., Öberg, M., Nielsen, C., Naylor, G., and Kramer, S., 2010. Factors influencing help seeking, hearing aid uptake, hearing aid use and satisfaction with hearing aids: a review of the literature. *Trends in Amplification*, 14(3), pp. 127–154.

Lupsakko, T., Kautiainen, H., and Sulkava, R., 2005. The nonuse of hearing aids in people aged 75 years and over in the city of Kuopio in Finland. *European Archive of Otorhinolaryngology*, 262, pp. 165–169.

Mahoney, C., Stephens, S., and Cadge, B., 1996. Who prompts patients to consult about hearing loss? *British Journal of Audiology*, 30(3), pp. 153–158.

Meyer, C. and Hickson, L., 2012. What factors influence help-seeking for hearing impairment and hearing aid adoption in older adults? *International Journal of Audiology*, 51(2), pp. 66–74.

Stephens, D. and Kramer, S., 2009. *Living with hearing difficulties: the process of enablement*. Chichester, West Sussex, UK: John Wiley & Sons, Ltd.

Tye-Murray, N., 1991. Repair strategy usage by hearing-impaired adults and changes following communication therapy. *Journal of Speech, Language, and Hearing Research*, 34(4), pp. 921–928.

Vinay and Moore, B., 2007. Speech recognition as a function of highpass filter cutoff frequency for subjects with and without low-frequency cochlear dead regions. *Journal of the Acoustical Society of America*, 122, pp. 542–553.

10

SELF-EVALUATION

Reflecting on experiences and whether rehabilitation has made a difference

Rebecca Kelly-Campbell

Introduction

The focus of this chapter is on self-evaluation following hearing rehabilitation. Hearing rehabilitation in this context includes amplification (i.e., hearing aids and other hearing assistive technology), instruction on effective communication, and counseling. It is important to note that there is an element of self-evaluation throughout the entire patient journey, from awareness to resolution. However, a person with hearing loss (PHL) tends to spend a significant amount of time trying to make meaning of hearing loss and reflecting on positive and negative aspects of hearing rehabilitation. The self-evaluation is heavily influenced by expectations and experiences of a PHL.

In evaluating the processes and outcomes of hearing rehabilitation, there are many different potential participants (see Figure 10.1). Additionally, many tools are readily available to assess these procedures and results. These include both objective and subjective assessments aimed at gaining understanding of the impact of hearing therapy for individuals. Another assessment option is for the PHL to make a *self-evaluation* of the rehabilitation. A PHL may ask themselves about their own perceptions of the influence of hearing therapy in their lives. These self-evaluations have been found to differ from evaluations by practitioners. In a qualitative study by Manchaiah et al. (2011), PHLs who wore hearing aids were asked about their journey and experiences with hearing loss. Practitioners were also asked about their perceptions of the patient's journey. Differences were exhibited when PHLs identified this self-evaluation aspect of the journey. Practitioners did not distinguish this self-evaluation category. However, this new theme is of great importance as self-evaluations may reveal new information not found in assessments made by others (e.g., practitioners, family members, friends, and colleagues). This relationship is shown in Figure 10.1. From a person-centered audiological rehabilitation (PCAR)

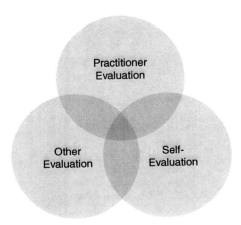

FIGURE 10.1 Different types of evaluations of outcomes of hearing rehabilitation

perspective, these self-evaluations are a vital part of understanding the journey of experiencing hearing loss.

This chapter mainly addresses the self-evaluation of the PHL and also its relation to evaluation by others. However, we do not discuss others' evaluation on its own in detail. Two case examples have been used to illustrate the dimensions of the self-evaluation phase. In one example there is more agreement in terms of self-evaluation of the PHL and evaluation by others when compared to the other example.

Further considering available tools to hearing healthcare practitioners for assessment of hearing rehabilitation outcomes, there is a variety available. One such tool is often used to objectively assess one part of hearing rehabilitation, amplification. Hearing healthcare practitioners often perform objective electroacoustic assessments of the function of the hearing aid. They use standardized procedures to ensure the devices are working appropriately and are providing the amplification specifications deemed appropriate for that individual. However, this type of evaluation only assesses the intervention at the *body level*, that is, at the level of the loss. Practitioners can also evaluate intervention at the *person* and *society levels*, that is, at the level of activity and participation, respectively. A common way to perform evaluations at these levels is through self-report questionnaires. Evaluation of intervention at person and society levels is an important aspect of PCAR, since the decision to seek audiological intervention is more strongly related to perceived difficulties of the PHL in activities and participation than with impairment (Swan and Gatehouse, 1990).

Since PHLs do not experience hearing loss in isolation (see Chapter 1), it is important to also assess the perception of communication partners (CPs) regarding outcomes of intervention. Note that the perception of the PHL and the CPs may not always be the same (see Chapters 3 and 4). In a study evaluating a group audiological rehabilitation program, Habanec and Kelly-Campbell (2015) found that, before hearing rehabilitation, PHLs and CPs had different perceptions of the

PHL's adjustment and communication functioning. Following intervention, CPs reported greater impact of hearing rehabilitation on their partners' adjustment and functioning than the PHLs reported. This exhibits how PHL and CP perceptions may differ at various stages in the patient journey. These findings further highlight the importance of exploring the self-evaluation by the PHL. However, as the findings of Manchaiah and colleagues (2011) indicated, practitioners do not necessarily identify self-evaluation as part of the patient journey.

Case examples

Two case examples are provided to demonstrate the concepts of self-evaluation in this chapter. The case examples are drawn from interviews about couples' experiences of hearing loss (Kelly-Campbell and Plexico, 2012). Some wording has been changed to preserve the anonymity of the patients.

Holly

Holly is a mother and homemaker. Holly and her husband, Gene, have two teenage children living at home. Holly experienced a sudden, permanent unilateral hearing loss following the identification and removal of a facial tumor. During the acute phase of her journey, Gene and the children were very supportive. After the acute phase of Holly's journey ended, Holly continued to face communication difficulties. Holly considered various hearing aid devices, including a bone-anchored hearing aid, which requires surgery. Holly's family was not supportive of that decision. Gene was worried about possible medical complications and did not perceive that Holly had difficulty with communication. Holly and Gene did not share the same perception about Holly's communication difficulties or how Holly's journey should take shape.

Mark

Mark is a retired dentist. He lives with his wife, Clara, who is also retired. Mark and Clara noticed a gradual decrease in his hearing and together consulted a physician about his hearing. After being referred for a hearing test, Mark and Clara decided to purchase a set of hearing aids. Clara attended follow-up appointments and a group class aimed at learning communication strategies for PHLs. Mark and Clara shared similar perceptions about Mark's communication difficulties and solutions for helping improve communication at home.

Process of self-evaluation

People's experiences can be examined before, during, and after hearing rehabilitation. Before hearing rehabilitation, a PHL may become aware of communication difficulties and move towards seeking help for hearing loss. The PHL may reflect on

TABLE 10.1 Main aspects related to getting used to hearing aids, which relate to the self-evaluation phase (adapted from Dawes et al., 2014)

Main aspects	Specific aspects
Adjusting to new sound	• Occlusion effect • Unnatural sound
Practical use	• Hearing aid comfort • Remembering hearing aids • Manipulating hearing aids • Cleaning and maintenance • Managing batteries
Experimenting with use	• Functioning: capacity vs. performance • Trying unilateral and bilateral amplification • Listening strategies • Experimenting hearing aids with TV, in cinema, while using telephone and listening to music • Evaluation of rehabilitation as a whole

Psychological factors	• Redefine self-identify
	• Redefine self-image
	  – Managing stigma
	  – Increased confidence
	• Broadened experiences
	• Expectations
	• Renegotiate communicative interactions

various experiences of communication and communication breakdowns. During hearing rehabilitation, the PHL may be focused on the processes of diagnosis and determining the most appropriate rehabilitation option. After hearing rehabilitation, the PHL may focus on self-evaluation.

As illustrated in Table 10.1, the literature on the PHL getting used to hearing rehabilitation (e.g., hearing aids) suggests a number of dimensions, including: adjusting to new sounds; practical use of devices; experimenting with use; and psychological factors (Dawes et al., 2014). In this chapter, some of the main factors in relation to experimenting with use and psychological factors will be discussed and illustrated with examples.

Meaning-making: self-image and self-identity

One part of the self-evaluation process may involve attempts to understand the hearing loss (Manchaiah et al., 2011). Since humans often attempt to make meaning of life events, PHLs may wonder why they have a hearing loss. People draw on past experiences and anticipation of future experiences to help them make meaning of and understand events in their lives (Kelly, 1955). This meaning-making exercise may influence a person's *self-image* and *self-identity*. Self-image can be thought of as a person's internal view of self. Self-identity can be thought of as a person's external view of self. These viewpoints can be viewed in the stigma attached to hearing loss. That stigma can be perceived as being focused internally (threatening self-image) or focused externally (threatening self-identity). The examples below further illustrate these concepts. Some wording has been altered for clarity or for anonymity of the patients involved.

Holly's meaning-making

Holly's sudden hearing loss caused her anxiety, as she had no prior experience with hearing difficulty from which to draw meaning and anticipate her communication functioning. Holly had difficulty making meaning of her experience and she described it as: "a shock to my system. I had no idea what was happening and how to deal with it." She described how the experience influenced her self-image: "I've always thought of myself as a young, healthy person. But now, I don't know." She also described how stigma affected her self-identity: "I'm really a competent person. But now, I feel like I'm losing my edge … I feel like I'm an old lady who can't keep up … I'm embarrassed to tell people about [my hearing] loss because they may think that I'm getting past it." Interestingly, Gene also commented on the stigma attached to hearing loss and how he chose not to disclose Holly's hearing loss: "People ask me what's wrong with [Holly]. I tell them 'nothing' … I'm not sure why, I guess it's just none of their business."

Mark's meaning-making

Mark did not show signs of anxiety associated with his hearing difficulties. Over the years of his declining hearing, he and Clara adopted strategies for dealing with communication breakdowns. Most notably, they used humor to diffuse situations. Mark commented that they "made a game of it. When I made a mistake, [Clara] would give me that look. Then, I knew I had it wrong." This strategy was in line with Mark's self-image as a person who "takes things in their stride. I don't let [things] get to me." Mark acknowledged there was stigma attached to hearing loss, but did not feel this threatened his self-image: "People say that's part of getting older. But, I am an older person – as long as I take care of it [hearing loss], it's not a problem." Clara shared that perception: "Sure, I suppose it's something you expect at our age … we can laugh about these things at our age."

These case examples show that Holly and Mark experienced their journey quite differently, which influenced their experiences of meaning-making. Holly's journey through awareness and movement was abrupt. Holly and her family struggled to make meaning of Holly's sudden hearing loss and to incorporate that information into their lives. As a result, Holly was not able to integrate her experience into her self-image or self-identity. Mark's journey through awareness and movement was much more gradual. He and his CP, Clara, worked together to make meaning of Mark's hearing loss. As a result, they were successfully able to assign reason for the hearing loss and to integrate their experiences into their self-image and self-identity.

Functioning: capacity and performance

As discussed in Chapter 2, the World Health Organization (WHO) has recognized contextual factors to be an important component in determining the experience of a person with a health condition (World Health Organization, 2001). The contextual factors include: environmental factors and personal factors. The environmental factors include a person's home and work life, relationships (e.g., immediate and extended family), friends, acquaintances, neighbors, community members, persons in positions of authority, and health professionals. In addition, the attitudes of these individuals, social norms, and policies can also be included under the environmental factors. These environmental factors can act as either barriers or facilitators.

The WHO describes *capacity* as a person's ability to carry out a task or action (i.e., activity). A person's capacity may be different from a person's actual performance (i.e., participation). *Performance* refers to how well the person carries out that task or activity in everyday life. When a person's performance is worse than capacity, there exists a barrier in the person's environment. When a person's performance is better than capacity, there exists a facilitator in the person's environment.

Holly's functioning

Throughout Holly's journey, she has experienced many environmental barriers. For example, Holly is acutely aware of the stigma attached to hearing loss and that prevents her from asking for environmental accommodations. Because she has no measurable hearing in one ear, she knows that she needs to arrange the communication environment so she can make the most of the hearing in her unaffected ear. However, Holly does not actively ask others to make that accommodation for her, saying that she does not "want to put anyone out" or "be a bother" to anyone, particularly her family. Gene's attitude towards Holly's hearing loss sometimes also serves as a barrier. Gene does not like for Holly to drive when they travel, which places Holly with her worse ear facing Gene, resulting in Holly being unable to hear and carry on conversations in the car.

Mark's functioning

Throughout Mark's journey, he has experienced many environmental facilitators. For example, Mark obtained a set of hearing aids, which enable him to hear soft sounds. He is able to carry out a conversation with Clara in situations that he would not have been able to without his hearing aids. Mark commented on how his hearing aids have helped him: "With the aids, I can watch TV with [Clara] and it's not a problem. Before, it was too loud for her and she would leave the room." Clara also serves as a facilitator for Mark. Clara attended a communication class and learned some strategies to help improve communication at home. She reported that she "gets [Mark's] attention now" before she talks to him and tries to "make sure we're not talking where there's too much noise."

The experiences of both Holly and Mark provide examples of how environmental and personal factors have affected their journeys. In Holly's case, these factors led to barriers in functioning. In Mark's case, these factors served as facilitators to functioning.

Expectations: under-estimation and over-estimation

Before undertaking a hearing rehabilitation option, a PHL may have certain expectations about the outcome. These expectations about the outcome of hearing rehabilitation are important in the self-evaluation process. A PHL may have unrealistic expectations that either under-estimate or over-estimate the amount of improvement in functioning that hearing rehabilitation will provide. Cox and Alexander (2000) found that new hearing aid owners, before obtaining their first hearing aids, tended to have high and unrealistic expectations about hearing aids. These unrealistic expectations can influence how a PHL and CPs view their journeys before, during, and after hearing rehabilitation.

Holly's expectations

Holly and Gene had unrealistic expectations for the bone-anchored hearing aid. Holly commented that they anticipated a "quick fix" for her hearing loss. They were both disappointed to learn that the bone-anchored hearing aid would not fully restore Holly's hearing. Neither Holly nor Gene explored any options other than the bone-anchored hearing aid. After opting out of the surgery, Holly commented on her lack of options: "That's about all we can do now."

Mark's expectations

Mark and Clara had reasonable expectations for their hearing rehabilitation. Mark commented that hearing aids "don't fix everything." As a result, he and Clara attended communication classes to learn strategies to improve functioning. As Mark explained: "The classes were set up to teach us how to get the most out of the aids."

Evaluation of rehabilitation: positive and negative

As shown by Manchaiah et al. (2011), a PHL may evaluate both positive and negative aspects of hearing rehabilitation. PHLs and CPs reflect on the positive and negative experiences throughout their journeys and try to assign reason for the hearing loss. This evaluation is a culmination of their meaning-making, functioning, and expectations of hearing rehabilitation. Experiences through these aspects affect the evaluation of hearing rehabilitation.

Holly's evaluation of rehabilitation

Holly described trying to assign reason for her hearing loss: "I don't know why this happened to me. I've always tried to live a healthy lifestyle." She reflected on the positive and negative aspects of a bone-anchored hearing aid: "It isn't going to help in every situation and they can have lots of complications ... There's just no guarantee that it'll help." She attributed her ultimate decision to reject the hearing aid in part on these reflections: "So [Gene] is probably right. It's not worth the risk."

Mark's evaluation of rehabilitation

Mark saw aging as the reason for his hearing loss: "It's what you would expect at my age." Mark and Clara both reflected on positive and negative experiences with hearing aids. Mark commented that the hearing aids "are a big help, especially at home." He continues to struggle to communicate in "noisy places" where the aids "don't work." Mark's decision to accept the hearing aids is likely due to the overall positive self-evaluation: "All in all, they are well worth it ... one of the best decisions we made."

While Holly was not able to assign reason for her hearing loss, Mark did. This may have contributed to the differences in their level of acceptance of the hearing loss. Holly mostly reflected on the negative aspects of her hearing rehabilitation option. In contrast, Mark mostly reflected on the positive aspects of his hearing rehabilitation.

Person-centered care: understanding and application

It is important for practitioners to understand these evaluations and their application to PCAR. In person-centered care (PCC), practitioners work collaboratively with patients to help identify treatment options. Manchaiah et al. (2011) demonstrated that while PHLs experienced self-evaluation, practitioners who work with PHLs did not recognize this aspect of the patient journey. Hence, practitioners should pay careful attention to the self-evaluation of PHLs as it may have important implications for their rehabilitation. To that end, practitioners should attempt to gain understanding about the PHLs' self-evaluation and tailor treatment options that suit the needs of the PHL.

Holly's person-centered care

Holly's self-evaluation indicated that she viewed her journey negatively. She continues to experience barriers to successful communication and restrictions in her social participation. Holly's journey began suddenly, and she was not able to make meaning of her hearing loss. Holly's experience resulted in negative self-image and self-identity. She had many environmental barriers and had unrealistically high expectations of bone-anchored hearing aids.

A PCC approach to Holly's journey might have resulted in a more positive outcome. PCC for Holly would focus on her attitudes towards her experience and work towards forming a more positive self-identity and self-image. This can be accomplished by providing Holly with information about hearing loss and treatment options and psychosocial support counseling. Inclusion of Holly's family in this process would be helpful. Holly and her family focused solely on the option of a bone-anchored hearing aid. A more PCC approach would also focus on other ways to improve Holly's communication performance. This can be accomplished by providing Holly and her CPs with information about Holly's communication performance and collaboratively finding non-surgical options to facilitate performance.

Mark's person-centered care

Mark's evaluation indicated he viewed his journey positively. Mark's journey began gradually, allowing Mark and Clara time to work through the meaning-making process before seeking treatment. Mark and Clara were ready to make behavioral changes when they encountered their practitioner. Mark experiences few barriers to communication and few restrictions in his social participation. Mark and Clara had realistic expectations about using hearing aids and enrolled in communication classes.

Mark and Clara were provided with support from their practitioner in the form of PCC. They worked collaboratively with their practitioner to set realistic goals and adopt a holistic approach to care. This included the provision of hearing aids as well as reducing environmental barriers and drawing on environmental facilitators.

Summary

This chapter focused on the self-evaluation that PHLs and CPs assume as part of their journey with hearing loss. These case studies of Holly and Mark highlight the importance of PCAR and PCC. Holly required more time to adjust to her hearing loss before making a decision about her rehabilitation options. Perhaps because of an environmental modifier (e.g., technocentric approach), Holly continues to experience significant ongoing communication difficulties and social isolation. Mark's journey was more person-centered and as a result, he and Clara experience little residual communication difficulties and have adjusted to the hearing loss.

Self-evaluation is an important part of the patient journey. Holly and Mark experienced different journeys, yet they both performed this self-evaluation in which they reflected on their experiences. Research shows that it is not likely that their practitioners recognize this important part of the journey. For Holly, careful attention to her self-evaluation could move her from continued communication difficulty and social withdrawal to successful communication and social participation.

References

Cox, R. and Alexander, G., 2000. Expectations about hearing aids and their relationship to fitting outcome. *Journal of the American Academy of Audiology*, 11, pp. 368–382.

Dawes, P., Maslin, M., and Munro, K., 2014. "Getting used to" hearing aids from the perspective of adult hearing-aid users. *International Journal of Audiology*, 53, pp. 861–870.

Habanec, O. and Kelly-Campbell, R., 2015. Outcomes of group audiological rehabilitation for unaided adults with hearing impairment and their significant others. *American Journal of Audiology*, 24, pp. 40–52.

Kelly, G., 1955. *The psychology of personal constructs.* New York, NY: Norton Publishing.

Kelly-Campbell, R. and Plexico, L., 2012. Couples' experiences living with hearing impairment. *Asia Pacific Journal of Speech Language, and Hearing*, 15, pp. 145–160.

Manchaiah, V., Stephens, D., and Meredith, R., 2011. The patient journey of adults with hearing impairment: the patients' view. *Clinical Otolaryngology*, 36, pp. 227–234.

Swan, I. and Gatehouse, S., 1990. Factors influencing consultation for management of hearing disability. *British Journal of Audiology*, 24, pp. 155–160.

World Health Organization, 2001. *International Classification of Functioning, Disability and Health (ICF)*. Geneva, Switzerland: World Health Organization.

11

RESOLUTION – PART 1

Recapturing the conversation – hearing loss and communication

Berth Danermark

Introduction

It is well known that the most important consequence of hearing loss is the reduced ability to communicate (Stephens et al., 1995). As discussed in Chapter 2, the reduced function in communication results in self-perception of hearing loss and forms the driving force for taking action to restore lost function. The next two chapters focus on the *resolution phase* of the journey through hearing loss. This phase includes the person with hearing loss (PHL) adapting and changing, considering social impact, considering cost and time, resolving or not resolving problems satisfactorily, and identifying new problems. This chapter will provide better understanding of the primary aspects of conversation. The following chapter will focus more on secondary and long-term aspects of living with hearing loss (e.g., depression and loneliness).

Restoring conversation and improving communication is the ultimate goal of audiological rehabilitation. To get an idea of what it means to acquire hearing loss and how it affects communication, it is helpful to have a general idea of what is involved in conversation, in particular how we make meaning of what is said. Conversation is an extremely complex social action. It requires well-developed social skills as well as hearing ability. Hence, the first part of the chapter is devoted to describing the principles of communication and conversation. The second part will address the question of what to do in order to recapture conversation and how to maintain the abilities necessary for communication. In this part, some common advice provided for communication will be covered and related to treatments discussed later in this chapter.

Communication is an umbrella term for a wide range of actions. One of a number of possible ways to communicate is to interact (Giles and Street, 1994). Interaction is action between people, such as conversing, which requires a minimum of two active parties. Other ways of communicating do not necessarily require this direct person-to-person relationship.

Why do we interact with other people? The question may seem strange to many. It can be regarded as so obvious that the question need not be asked. It is posed here because the answers may vary greatly because there are different reasons why we interact. Some claim that it has to do, primarily, with *satisfying our needs*. Interaction, in this case, is seen as an instrumental activity: We interact because we want to accomplish or achieve something. Others maintain that we interact to create meaning in life. This aim of interaction is thus termed the *creation of meaning*. Still others say that the aim of interaction is social: It serves to give us a place in social life, to establish and maintain *social relationships*. Interaction can serve all three of these aims, though here the two latter approaches will be stressed with greater emphasis on social relationships (Grossberg, 1982).

Conversation

This section focuses on conversation as an action performed together with others. One *con*-verses, that is, speaks together with one or more people. It may also be viewed as a form of *co*-operation, a talking together about something. The latter means that we endeavor to understand one another, to create a common meaning or sense in the flow of words. This is the essence of conversation – the joint creation of meaning. This means that conversation can be seen as a process, a dialogue, something that requires the active participation of both parties, and it is in this process that understanding emerges (see Linell, 1998).

Another common way of looking at conversation is to consider the sender, message, and receiver. We can think of a meteorologist who presents the weather on radio or television. They have a well-prepared "message" that they "send." The "receiver," sitting at home, "receives" the message. The hope is that the message sent will arrive and be understood in the way it was intended. However, the "sending" can be disturbed or disrupted (e.g., technical difficulties) so that the message does not arrive intact. Furthermore, the content of the message may be too complicated for the listener to understand, or there could be interference in the listening environment (e.g., noise from neighbors), which results in the message not fully reaching the receiver. This way of looking at communication is relevant in many situations, such as the one described above. When analyzing communication such as conversation, this method has proved insufficient. It simply does not capture the "meaning-making" process that is the essence of conversation.

In the following section, five different aspects of conversation will be highlighted. The first is that conversation is a flow of utterances, and the order of these utterances is significant: *sequence* is central. Second, a conversation is always about something. The utterances occur in a *context*. A third aspect of conversation is that it is a *joint meaning-making process*. It is not the case that an individual gives an utterance meaning. This is done together. Fourth, in conversation, we distribute this meaning-making work (*the division of labor*) among the conversation's participants. The fifth and final aspect is that body language, tone, and other types of "gestures" are very important. These are sometimes called a conversation's *metalanguage*.

Sequence

A conversation happens sequentially. This means that a statement is interpreted and understood in relation to other statements either preceding or following it. This can be illustrated with a brief story about John.

BOX 11.1

- John is on his way to school.
- He is worried about the math lesson.
- Last week, he had not been able to keep order in the classroom.
- It wasn't nice of the teacher to give him the assignment of keeping the class quiet all by himself.
- It isn't part of a custodian's normal duties.

What this simple example shows is that as we receive new information, we must reinterpret what has been said earlier. This is the first lesson we can learn from the example: When we hear something, we automatically put it into context. If the context is not given, we "make one up." We might assume that John is a student.

The second statement, "he is worried about the math lesson," does not challenge our first interpretation, but rather, reinforces it – it must be a troubled student on his way to school. However, then comes something that interferes with our interpretation, "Last week he had not been able to keep order in class." This statement may challenge our initial interpretation. Many reinterpret the first two statements and "understand" that John might be a newly qualified teacher or a teacher with a new class, or something similar.

Now, assume that we have not heard the third statement correctly, and still think that John is a student while all others understand him to be a teacher. In this situation, a person might very well make a comment that seems very strange to others.

Then comes the fourth statement, "It wasn't nice of the teacher to give him the assignment of keeping the class quiet all by himself." This statement may further challenge our interpretation. We must reinterpret everything that was said all over again. Perhaps it is a teacher in training, or is it a student who is prefect of the class? This raises some uncertainty for the person who is hard of hearing. "Did I miss something? Who is John?" In other words, is my uncertainty due to what was actually said, or is it because of my hearing loss? If the lack of clarity is due to the statement itself, then it is natural to ask for clarification. However, if I believe that everyone else has a clear picture and it is just me who does not "follow," then I am faced with the difficult choice of whether to ask or pretend to understand.

Finally, the last statement comes: "It isn't part of a custodian's normal duties." It seems simple, but what we may not realize is that we have again conducted an extremely complex and demanding intellectual operation, a reinterpretation of a series of different statements.

Not much reflection is required to understand that key words must be heard in order to get the full meaning of a conversation. A person who missed any of the previous statements may have difficulty following the story. This example illustrates the principles of conversation. Turns succeed one another, and interpretations shift. A person must be "up to date" with the right interpretation before they speak. Otherwise, they might come across as strange or different. How does one stay "up to date" if one is unsure, because of hearing loss, of having heard everything? As a rule, the choice is between asking for clarification and guessing.

Asking has its advantages and disadvantages. Among the advantages, of course, is that asking reduces the risk of further confusion due to misinterpretation. The disadvantages, however, are many. There are social limits to how often one can ask for clarification. One can ask at most two or three times before reaching a socially defined limit. It rarely makes sense to ask for clarification when jokes or funny stories are being told. There are also other limits with regard to asking. An important part of conversation is a natural flow, or *fluency*. To repeatedly interrupt this flow with "what?" or "huh?" can be disturbing and annoying to others, which they often cannot hide (Gangé and Willy, 1989).

The second choice, to guess, also has its pros and cons. If one guesses correctly, it works, but if not, embarrassing situations can occur. In certain types of conversations, one simply cannot guess (e.g., a nurse talking to a doctor about a patient cannot afford to guess what the doctor is saying).

Context

Many people with hearing loss are incredibly good at guessing. This may be because they can put the fragments of words heard in the right context. Consider *low predictable* and *highly predictable* words. For instance, in the sentence "She heard a growl," the word "growl" has low predictability because there is no context. However, in the sentence "The dog made a low growl," the word "growl" is highly predictable.

In certain situations, a change of context is clearly signaled. For example, in a television news program, the camera angle changes, the newscaster switches to a different sheet of paper in front of her, etc. This is done to mark the transition to a new subject. In more everyday contexts, however, such clear indications are unusual.

Consider another situation when two conversations are going on in parallel. While this may be unusual for some, for many it is typical to talk about two different things at once.

Joint meaning-making

Thus far, we have discovered how we create meaning by interpreting statements in relation to other statements and by understanding the context in which they are uttered. This may give the impression that the creation of meaning is an individual act. It is not. The creation of meaning is, as mentioned, a *co*-creation. We do it together with the people with whom we *con*verse. A *con*versation is characterized by those *con*versing having the aim to establish a common meaning. This is central.

When my communication partner (CP) uses an expression I do not understand, I ask what it means. She explains the meaning and checks with me to make sure I have understood. Periodically, she asks, "Are you following me?" and I nod (if I think I understand). If I am uncertain, I ask, "So you mean …?" In this way, we have a *con*versation, and a common meaning is established. If we think about it, this is the way a conversation is usually conducted, with interpolations, questions, comments, and body language. We are continually signaling that we follow.

The division of labor

The creation of meaning in normal everyday conversation is a joint action; it requires action by both parties. In order to function, it requires that both take responsibility. The question is then how this responsibility and work is distributed. How it is distributed in practice may vary from case to case depending on a number of different conditions (e.g., experience and knowledge). Most essential is that those involved experience symmetry in the work required for the conversation to function. If one partner feels that the other does not assume proper responsibility or "make an effort," an imbalance results, negatively affecting the relationship. In a couple's relationship, this can lead to unnecessary tension and discord. This can be avoided by raising the issue of the distribution of work and coming to an agreement about a distribution that both feel is practical and fair.

As the task is common to both parties, it is incumbent upon the PHL to assume his or her responsibility. This means, for example, that upon a deterioration in hearing, the PHL goes to the audiology clinic, takes an active part in the rehabilitation services offered, and uses technical aids made available to him or her. It also entails informing others about what works and what does not work, when one hears and when one does not hear, to name a few examples. The CP should assume his or her responsibility as well. For example, there are a wide range of practical issues to be aware of, including but not limited to: not talking with your mouth full or keeping your hand away from the mouth, not turning away when speaking, or not standing in front of a stark light.

It is easy to say that both should take responsibility, but it is sometimes difficult to do. There are many counteracting forces (Danermark et al., 1999). A person may have difficulty accepting his or her acquired hearing loss. And what does it mean to "accept one's responsibility?" Experience within audiological rehabilitation shows that it is important that this occurs at a pace the hard of hearing person can handle. As illustrated in several chapters in this book (e.g., Chapters 6 and 7), it can take many years of internal struggle before a PHL reaches a state of acceptance such that he or she can assume his or her part of the responsibility. Another counteracting force is the general nature of others' treatment or reception of people with hearing loss. If it is negative, then the PHL might want to avoid wearing a hearing aid or to let it be known that he or she has a hearing loss. Even here, it might be considered what is reasonable to expect of the person with hearing loss. These examples show that accountability is a complex issue. There are no easy answers to the questions raised. The expectations one can have of a PHL must be based upon prevailing conditions so that the person can contribute his or her part to the effort needed to make the conversation work.

If we now consider the CP, there correspond a number of counteracting forces. The first and perhaps most important hinder is that it is very difficult to change one's way of speaking. From the moment we are born and throughout our early years, we are encouraged to converse in a certain way. This conversational behavior is then continually reinforced throughout life. In our manner of speaking, we concentrate on what we regard as most important, on *what* we will say. *How* we say it is something we do without being fully aware of it. For a short time, we can concentrate on both how and what, but our concentration on how disappears very quickly over time.

When it comes to the question of an equitable division of labor in order for the conversation to work, there are thus great difficulties. To accept the responsibility does not automatically entail that it works. In hearing rehabilitation, one often gains very good knowledge and understanding about how to converse. This knowledge is necessary, but insufficient.

In sum, the purpose of this section has been to highlight a different type of knowledge: awareness of the necessity to strike a workable balance in the allocation of work in getting the conversation to function, with equal insight into the serious difficulties this involves.

Metalanguage

Conversation also contains other signals, such as pauses, emphases, and tempo. All of these aspects are indispensable as we interpret and give meaning to what is said (Burgoon, 1994). When we cannot follow a conversation, it can usually be seen in our faces. The movements are small, but the slightly wrinkled brow or questioning look shows that we are not really following. That the signals are often subtle, yet recognizable, is exemplified by the phrase "the questioning look." It is easy for us to recognize, but hard to describe.

With the body, we thus signal a great number of things that are needed in order for the conversation to go well. As indicated above, the face is an important window to our CPs. There we show compassion or indifference, joy or sorrow, pride or guilt, appreciation or irritation. Our facial expression can also be confirmatory or questioning. It can signal recognition or unfamiliarity.

With our eyes and our bodies, we can also signal, "I do not want to talk to you." This is also something that the hard of hearing sometimes experience. People in their surroundings are reluctant to converse, and it is signaled clearly through body language.

Furthermore, the way we speak carries information that we have learned to interpret. Many times, this occurs unconsciously. It is so programmed in us that we do not think about it. How is it, for example, that turn-taking works? How does one know when someone's contribution (turn) is ending so that someone else can come in with his or her contribution, or turn? This can be signaled in various subtle ways: with the eyes (the speaker may look up at the CPs in a clearer way), or with the voice (micro pauses between words change slightly, the tone changes). If a person does not perceive all of these subtle signals and "cannot keep up," it is easy to be left out of the conversation.

Another feature of the language is how words are emphasized differently, and what kind of emotional charge we give them. If a person fails to perceive these word tones, this can easily lead to misunderstanding.

What to do in order to recapture the lost conversation?

Following are a variety of things that can be done to help the situation.

A set of rules for how to behave in order to facilitate conversations is therefore usually provided in the rehabilitation context. These are:

BOX 11.2 Practical tips for the persons with hearing loss

- Speak clearly yourself – it is contagious!
- Practice lip reading.
- Listen with concentration – but relax sometimes!
- Take it easy if difficulties arise in the conversation. Use humor!
- Accept hearing loss as something you certainly do not need to be ashamed of.
- Always place yourself with the light behind you so that the light falls on your CP.
- Address others only when you are close enough to surely be able to hear the reply.

- It is better not to respond at all when someone speaks to you from another room, if you do not hear what is said.
- Tell others what your hearing loss entails.
- Let people know that you are not disinterested if you do not answer, but that it is because you have not heard.
- Remember that the hearing loss is not the whole person. Behind it is the essential, the unique personality, always worth getting to know, believing in and developing.

Sometimes these guidelines are perceived as difficult to follow because they infringe on our habitual way of speaking.

Box 11.3 Practical tips for communication partners (e.g., relatives and work colleagues)

- Learn about hearing impairment and how you should speak for best results.
- Get the hearing impaired person's attention before you speak.
- Do not stand too far away or in another room when you speak.
- Turn your face toward the hard of hearing person and make sure your face is in the light.
- Do not stand with your back to the light.
- Do not hold your hand in front of your mouth when you speak.
- Speak with natural movements of the mouth – lip reading is a good support for many.
- Speak in your normal voice; do not shout.
- Make sure that one person talks at a time.
- Correct misunderstandings and repeat those things your conversational partner did not catch right away.
- Repeat and write down particularly important information and tasks.
- Do not change the subject of the conversation without warning.
- Enunciate technical terms and new words extra clearly.

These rules are relatively easy to learn, though their observance can be quite taxing. In the following, some conversational behaviors will be highlighted that may be more complicated to manage than the relatively simple rules listed above.

The first is how to make sure that the joint creation of meaning works and happens in a coordinated manner so that both take responsibility for it. The second behavior has to do with how one maintains the important flow of conversation. In practice, these two aspects of conversation are very closely linked. To ask for clarification with a "huh?", for example, is precisely to request assistance in the creation of meaning. I will still treat the two aspects separately, but it should be kept in mind that in everyday conversation they are intertwined.

The guidelines listed above are no guarantee that the conversation will go smoothly. They can be seen as necessary but insufficient conditions.

Pay attention to the creation of meaning

The basic rule for a successful conversation is to *pay attention to the creation of meaning*. It can be a constant strain to try to follow and participate in a conversation. Because the person with normal hearing generally experiences the creation of meaning in a conversation as unproblematic, it is the CPs who most often fall short in this respect. To pay attention to the creation of meaning involves being aware and attentive to it in a completely different way. Suddenly the importance of all the little signals that indicate that someone is following or that they have a problem are visible.

However, you might choose another option, to continue talking and leave it to the PHL to ask when he or she does not hear or if something is unclear. If you do this consistently, this means that you are evading the PHL's responsibility for the creation of meaning. An asymmetry arises, undermining the relationship in the end.

Finding the right balance

The problem is to find the right balance between the two alternatives. Constantly making sure that the other person is following the conversation can easily be perceived as infantilizing – clearly not how one wants to be treated as an adult. It may also be the case that the conversation takes place in a context in which not all are aware that the person in question has a hearing loss. In this case, if you stop to ensure that he or she is following, then you are the one letting on to the others that he or she has a hearing loss. You do not let him or her decide for himself or herself if he or she wants to tell others in this particular context about his or her hearing loss. Yet, another reason not to constantly ask him or her if he or she "follows" is that what is said is not always important. The problem is that the other cannot decide whether it is important or not if he or she has not understood what was said.

Personal responsibility

The PHL must also assume his/her part of the responsibility and be clear in her actions. It is not just about signaling when one has *not* understood. It is at least as important to continually confirm that *one is following* the conversation, for example, by nodding or by other typical expressions for communicating that one has understood what has been said. Now this sounds easy, but it can be quite complicated in all the different contexts in which one participates in a conversation. There is a limit to how often and how obviously one wants to demonstrate that one has understood everything that has been said. This limit depends on the context. In small talk around the coffee table, with a constant buzz of background voices, it is perhaps not so important to understand everything, as compared to in a family meeting about an upcoming vacation.

Conversations of another type take place in more formal and official contexts. Such a conversation might be, for example, a meeting of an association or an information meeting at work. Here, the PHL must often embrace a different strategy. He or she can, for example, go through the most important points afterwards with one of the other participants.

Clear turn-taking benefits all

As shown, a conversation consists of turns and turn-taking. For a more in-depth discussion of this, see *Communication Therapy for Adults with Sensory Loss*, by Norman P. Erber (1996), especially chapter 8. See also *Communication and Adult Hearing Loss*, by Norman P. Erber (1993). What was termed "lines" above can also be called "turns." To hold a conversation is to periodically "take a turn," so to speak. For a PHL, this can be an especially trying situation. In a two-part conversation, it is not usually a major problem, although even in these conversations uncertainties may occur. In general, the problem arises when there are more than two people involved in the conversation. One way of facilitating such conversations is to not talk at the same time, which may be hard to resist. It is part of the dynamic of informal conversations that they are filled with occurrences of interjections and interruptions – that people "jump in" or cut others short.

There is a limit, however, to controlling informal conversations so that they are optimal for a PHL. If this limit is exceeded, the conversation will no longer be experienced as living, but can almost take on the character of a committee meeting. The difficulty lies in finding the right balance where everyone takes responsibility such that each person in the group may participate in the conversation. There is an important point to this approach, and this is that it not only benefits people who have difficulty following a group conversation because of their hearing. It also benefits those who find it difficult to jump into a conversation, those who are not as "pushy" as others or who tend to consider their words more carefully.

Such a manner of conversing in groups is characterized in part by the fact there are clear turn-taking markers. By this I mean that the person who speaks more clearly than usual signals that "now I am finished with what I've been saying," or "now I want to come into the conversation," and so on. Conversation is also facilitated by clear, non-verbal signals, such as body language that underlines what one is saying and/or that one is following the conversation.

In sum, all that was discussed in this section has to do with jointly distributing the work of making the conversation flow. A few practical solutions were provided, but the list can be made much longer. It is all about being aware of the difficulties and the importance of how a person converses to then take the plunge and put knowledge into practice.

ICF and conversation

Impeded conversation is the most often mentioned consequence of hearing loss by PHL. This was shown in Chapter 2, when describing the results of the preparatory studies for the creation of ICF Core Sets for PHL, that it was the issue that the PHL themselves brought to the forefront, even though it was less frequent in research. This indicates a further need to focus more on this aspect of hearing loss. Furthermore, most of the categories regarding Activities & Participation and Environmental factors in the Brief Core Set for PHL are relevant for conversation, which indicates the importance of this aspect.

Summary

Perhaps the most important message of this chapter is that this is a task that must be shared in solidarity in the end. For many, it is a demanding task, which requires both insight and training. It often takes a long time to change one's manner of conversing. Some of the easier things to change are not standing against a light background, not conversing with one's hand in front of one's mouth, and speaking clearly. It is more difficult to change the very way one converses. Consider some of the ways it might need to be changed: (1) how to ask and answer when someone has not heard or fully understood what was said; (2) how to find the right balance between spontaneous conversation and more orderly conversation when speaking one on one; and (3) conversing in such a way that one is clear in one's turn-taking and body language. Finally yet importantly is the need to manage one's emotions – feelings that others do not care, irritability, resignation, and alienation, and even perhaps the CP's irritation and difficulty in understanding the situation.

References

Burgoon, J., 1994. Nonverbal signals. In Mark L. Knapp and Gerald R. Miller (Eds.), *Handbook of interpersonal communication*. London, UK: Sage Publishing.

Danermark, B., Collgård, J., and Fredriksson, C., 1999. *Dialogue analysis: A new method for evaluating audiological rehabilitation*, Report 4. Ahlséns Research Institute. Örebro, Sweden: Örebro University and University Hospital in Örebro.

Erber, N., 1993. *Communication and adult hearing loss*. Melbourne, Australia: Clavis Publishing.

Erber, N., 1996. *Communication therapy for adults with sensory loss*. Melbourne, Australia: Clavis Publishing.

Gangé, J.-P. and Willy, K., 1989. Relative effectiveness of three repair strategies on the visual-identification of misperceived words. *Ear and Hearing*, 10, pp. 368–374.

Giles, H. and Street, R., 1994. Communicator characteristics and behaviour. In Mark L. Knapp and Gerald R. Miller (Eds.), *Handbook of interpersonal communication*. London, UK: Sage Publishing, 2nd edition, pp. 103-161.

Grossberg, L., 1982. Does communication theory need intersubjectivity? Toward an immanent philosophy of interpersonal relations. In Michael Burgoon (Ed.), *Communication yearbook 6*. Beverly Hills, CA: Sage Publishing, pp. 171–205.

Linell, P., 1998. *Approaching dialogue: Talk, interaction and contexts in dialogical perspectives*. Philadelphia, PA: Amsterdam Publishing.

Stephens, D., France, L., and Lormore, K., 1995. Effects of hearing impairment on the patient's family and friends. *Acta Oto-laryngologica*, 155, pp. 165–167.

12

RESOLUTION – PART 2

Continuing to adapt to and live with hearing loss

Marieke Pronk, Mariska Stam, and Sophia E. Kramer

Introduction

As mentioned in previous chapters, this chapter focuses on continuing and adapting to live with hearing loss by discussing what can be learned from two large-scale ongoing Dutch cohort studies about psychosocial health consequences of hearing loss.

Findings from epidemiological studies can be used to learn if and to what extent the "average" person with hearing loss (PHL) is affected. In addition, they can be used to discover if there are subgroups of persons who seem to be affected more heavily by hearing loss than others. Two studies that are used for these purposes are described in this chapter: the Netherlands Longitudinal Study on Hearing (NL-SH) and the Longitudinal Aging Study Amsterdam (LASA). Before these findings are discussed, some case examples of how PHLs experience hearing disability in their daily lives are provided, thereby illustrating how this impacts their psychosocial health.

The impact of hearing loss – case examples

Following are the quotations from participants in a focus group (see Granberg et al., 2014). Names have been altered for privacy purposes.

Susannah

> I really do tend to withdraw [from social activities] … but sometimes others come and pick me up to do things, so I have to come … Then I'm worn out when I get home, it costs me so much effort … When I was younger, I didn't notice so much, but now I get older, it costs more energy […] You pull back a little bit, you become a bit insecure [because of hearing loss]. And the older you get, the more this seems to be prominent … It [the hearing loss] didn't

bother me so much when I was younger, but now I think "Oh …" […]
I would have loved taking courses in English, or painting. But I don't have the
guts. Then people go and talk to me and then I think: "Oh God." No, then
I'd rather not … You are a bit anxious. […]

(Susannah, 67 years old (profound hearing loss since childhood))

Louis

I tried to stop those little devices [hearing aids] for years, because I felt like,
yes, you immediately become an old man when you do that. But once I had
decided it for myself and I also told others, all I got were positive reactions.
People think it's a really good thing that you do it. That I really found striking.

*(Louis, 62 years old (moderate hearing loss since
13 years old, has worn hearing aids for six months))*

Anne

I am often irritated by people not willing to repeat or talk more slowly, and
sometimes I am depressed. Then I think: "My goodness." Yes, sometimes I am
depressed, because I can't hear well.

(Anne, 55 years old (moderate hearing loss for 20 years))

Jake

The social disability that any hearing-impaired person must experience, I'm
afraid, yes, I recognize those. That's major …

(Jake, 42 years old (mild hearing loss for six years))

The statements above provide a brief but typical range of experiences of how the
lives of PHLs can be affected by hearing difficulties. Social isolation or loneliness,
depression, insecurity or low self-esteem, and anxiety all are outcomes of what is
often referred to as poor "psychosocial health". This may result from the inability to
effectively adapt to, or cope with, hearing decline and its consequences on daily life
activities and social life (Andersson et al., 1996).

Jake, Anne, and Susannah suggest that their psychosocial health is affected negatively by their hearing loss, but how common is this among other PHLs? Does hearing loss affect PHLs equally? The answers is – not surprisingly – no. Not everyone is
affected, and among those who are, the impact varies across persons, and may even
vary from day to day. The degree of experienced disability and in this case, negative
emotions and mood, depend on the person, their physical and social environment,
and their interactions with the environment (see Chapter 1), the latter of which as
was already acknowledged by Noble and Hétu (1994). Formulated in the nomen-
clature of the International Classification of Functioning, Disability and Health
(ICF; World Health Organization, 2001), experienced disability is influenced by

contextual factors both internal to the person (e.g., demographic characteristics such as age and gender, and use of coping strategies) and external to the person (e.g., the social context and the acoustical listening environments a person is often in). There are individual differences, but what can be said about the relationship between hearing loss and psychosocial health *in general*, so for the average (older) adult? To answer this question epidemiological studies are needed.

Hearing epidemiology: principles and two examples of prospective cohort studies

Epidemiology is "the science that investigates the pattern of diseases in populations, to help understand both their causes and the burden they impose" (Bhopal, 2002). In the context of this chapter, it means that epidemiologists are interested in the consequences of hearing loss on psychosocial health outcomes. Typically, epidemio-logical studies involve large samples of participants in whom all sorts of relevant factors (e.g., hearing, psychosocial outcomes, demographic factors) are measured through standardized questionnaires or physical, functional performance tests. With statistical models, epidemiologists investigate whether, *on average*, PHLs experience more feelings of loneliness than people without hearing loss, and whether a dose response relationship exists when persons with mild hearing loss are compared to persons with more severe hearing loss. Epidemiologists usually adjust models for factors that bias the relationship or modify the relationship (e.g., different effects for men and women).

Different study designs exist. There are experimental and observational designs. In the latter, the investigator does not intervene but simply observes and measures the strength of the relationship between an "exposure variable" (degree of hear-ing problems in our case) and a "disease variable" (psychosocial health outcomes). Although various types of observational designs exist, in this chapter we will focus on the prospective cohort study design.

Prospective observational cohort studies follow groups of participants over a longer period of time. This provides unique knowledge in that the course of hear-ing ability in relation to a range of outcome variables (e.g., change in psychological, social, and emotional functioning), but also biasing factors (e.g., comorbid condi-tions) can be investigated. In addition, a longitudinal design allows researchers to incorporate a so-called "temporal relationship" criterion: the degree of exposure (e.g., hearing loss) can be identified before the outcome (e.g., psychosocial health) occurs. This implies that the results would provide strong scientific evidence for hearing loss indeed *causing* (preceding) poorer psychosocial health.

Netherlands Longitudinal Study on Hearing

In 2006, the NL-SH commenced (see Table 12.1). The NL-SH is an ongoing pro-spective cohort study. It is implemented via the internet. It is a unique cohort in that

TABLE 12.1 Study characteristics of the Netherlands Longitudinal Study on Hearing (NL-SH) and the Longitudinal Aging Study Amsterdam (LASA)

	Netherlands Longitudinal Study on Hearing (NL-SH)	Longitudinal Aging Study Amsterdam (LASA)
General aim of the study	Examine the long-term relationship between hearing ability* and various aspects of functioning in daily life.	Examine the predictors and consequences of changes in wellbeing in aging older adults.
Focus	Psychosocial health, work situation, use of health care.	Physical (including hearing ability*), psychosocial, cognitive, and social functioning.
Age of participants at the start of the study	18 to 70 years	55 to 85 years
Sample and administration mode	Convenience; online.	Population-based; face-to-face interviews at the respondents' homes.
Measurements over time	Baseline (2006), 5-year follow-up (2011), 10-year follow-up (2016), and ongoing.	Baseline (1992/1993) and since then every 3–4 years, and ongoing.

*Measured both by self-report and the digit triplet speech-in-noise test.

hearing disability is the central topic under investigation. The study sample consists of both adults with and without hearing loss, covering a wide age range. Hearing status is determined by an online hearing test, the Dutch digit triplet speech-in-noise test (Smits et al., 2004). It determines the ability of a person to recognize speech in background noise. This particular feature of hearing is relevant, as problems in this domain are central to age-related hearing loss, they are the most prevalent hearing complaint of PHLs. The NL-SH measurement battery further contains validated scales on socioeconomic status, health, self-reported hearing and hearing devices, psychosocial health status, participation in paid work and other domains of social life, and use of health care.

Longitudinal Aging Study Amsterdam

LASA is an on going cohort study on predictors and consequences of changes in autonomy and wellbeing in an aging population (Hoogendijk et al., 2016). It differs from the NL-SH in that hearing disability per se is not the central topic under study, but rather *one* of the health measures collected and investigated in this broad study on aging. LASA only includes older adults (55+ years). The first cycle of data collection was in 1992/1993 in a random sample of 3107 older persons (55 to 85 years) that was drawn from the Dutch municipality registers. In LASA, respondents are interviewed in their homes by trained interviewers and the same measurements are repeated every three to four years. A range of psychosocial, physical, cognitive, and demographical outcomes are assessed using standardized questionnaires and physical and cognitive performance tests. Hearing ability is assessed using self-report. Since the 2001/2002 measurement, also the Dutch digit triplet speech-in-noise test (the same as in the NL-SH) is included.

Psychosocial health effects of hearing loss – evidence from epidemiological studies

An abundant number of epidemiological studies have shown that the sum of disabilities that PHLs experience can seriously impact their psychosocial health. This chapter focuses on feelings of loneliness and depressive symptoms. These negative outcomes can be viewed as expressions of negative affect or mood, which are the result of long-lasting pressure on emotional functioning. The relevance of emotional functions for PHLs is underlined by the fact that they are part of the ICF Core Sets for Hearing Loss (ICF category b152: Emotional functions, see Appendix).

Emotional and social loneliness

Hearing loss can potentially cause disruption of close and more distant personal relations and cause an unmet need to fulfill desired social roles in a satisfactory way. On a more basic level, during conversations PHLs can feel left out because they are not able to participate fully in the conversation. These disabilities can potentially contribute to feelings of loneliness.

Loneliness is the subjective notion of experiencing an unpleasant or inadmissible lack of certain relationships or in the quality of certain relationships. Two components of loneliness can be distinguished. *Emotional loneliness* relates to a felt absence of a deep, or intimate relationship one usually has with a partner or a best friend. *Social loneliness* relates to experiencing deficits in social integration and embeddedness so concerns one's broader social network of siblings, cousins, friends, neighbors, and peers (e.g., see De Jong Gierveld, 1998).

In terms of (objective) social isolation, previous studies have shown that PHLs have smaller social networks, and hearing loss particularly hampers starting new relationships. In terms of subjective feelings of loneliness, most studies – some of which had a longitudinal study design – showed a significant relationship between hearing loss and a general measure of loneliness, although some other studies found no significant relationship. Up until 2011, studies with a longitudinal design that distinguished between emotional and social loneliness, were absent. In addition, possible subgroup-specific effects were hardly investigated. It was attempted to specifically address these gaps in evidence by analyzing the data of NL-SH and LASA.

Findings from NL-SH and LASA

The degree of hearing disability (as measured by self-report or the digit triplet speech-in-noise test) and social and emotional loneliness were prospectively associated, but moderately (see Table 12.2). On average, persons with relatively greater hearing disability had poorer scores on both measures of loneliness as compared to people with no or less hearing disability. Contrary to the NL-SH sample in which this effect was found in the total sample, a significant association appeared in specific subgroups of older persons only in the LASA respondents (Pronk et al., 2011). Only for men, those living with a partner, and non-hearing aid users was hearing disability associated with emotional or social loneliness.

Gender differences in the use of coping mechanisms may explain the adverse effect on emotional loneliness that was found only for men. Generally, men tend to use nonverbal communication strategies somewhat less often and report somewhat less problem awareness and more denial than women do (e.g., Garstecki and Erler, 1999). This in turn could add to worse coping with hearing problems and affecting the quality of close relationships negatively. With regard to social relations, men are generally more likely to find an intimate attachment figure in marriage, whereas women also find deep or intimate relationships with other close ties such as a good friend. It is likely that hearing loss places such a burden on close relations that men's experienced deficit becomes especially apparent when living with a partner

TABLE 12.2 The effects of hearing disability on social and emotional loneliness found in the Netherlands Longitudinal Study on Hearing (NL-SH) and the Longitudinal Aging Study Amsterdam (LASA)

Determinant	Outcome of interest	Sample	NL-SH	LASA
Hearing disability*	Emotional loneliness	Total sample	✓	✗
		Subgroup: Men	✗	✓
		Subgroup: Non-hearing aid users	✗	✓
		Subgroup: Living with partner in the household	–	✓
	Social loneliness	Total sample	✓	✗
		Subgroup: Non-hearing aid users	✗	✓
		Subgroup: Living with partner in the household	–	✓

* Measured by self-report or the digit triplet speech-in-noise test. For the purpose of simplicity the findings in this table are not further specified.
✓ Effect was tested and was present (statistically significant).
✗ Effect was tested and was not present (not statistically significant).
– Subgroup effect was not investigated, as partner status was not measured.

in the household. This is in line with previous evidence from studies convincingly showing that hearing loss can place a heavy burden on the partner relationship of the PHL, i.e., so-called third-party disability. Mutual irritation and frustration, a less personal relationship with loss of intimate talk and limited physical and emotional intimacy all are well-documented in couples in which one of the partners is hearing-impaired. This may also explain why in LASA it was found that particularly those living with a partner experienced more social loneliness due to hearing problems. With regard to the effect on *social* loneliness, it could be that PHLs compare themselves more strongly to their socially, relatively well-functioning partners than would be the case if a PHL lived alone, subsequently leading to stronger experiences of deficits in social embedding.

Lastly, the LASA findings suggest beneficial psychosocial effects of amplification through hearing aids. A significant effect on emotional and social loneliness was found for non-hearing aid users, while no adverse effects emerged for hearing aid users. The findings should be interpreted with caution though, as respondents were only asked whether they "*usually* used a hearing aid." The users could thus only represent the more satisfied, successful users. The findings nonetheless are in accordance with results of previous studies, which showed an association between hearing aid use, reduced hearing disability, and improvement in quality of life.

Depression

As described, hearing loss can disrupt communication abilities, personal relationships, and social roles, subsequently leading to loneliness. Each of these consequences could also contribute to depressed mood. According to the widely used theory on depression, a depressed mood is influenced by recurrent or automatic thoughts with negative content. Depressed persons both attend more to negative events in their lives more strongly as compared to non-depressed persons, and interpret events in light of their "dysfunctional" negative cognitions.

Negative emotions could also arise from restrictions that are not directly linked to communication. Examples are reduced enjoyment of listening to music, theatre, watching TV, or even of sound in itself. Further, depressed mood may stem from the notion of "getting old" and the experience of loss of physical function in general. The latter is often accompanied by grief and associated emotions of anger, denial, sadness, frustration, loss of control, low self-worth, and embarrassment. Many studies found a significant association between hearing status and depressive symptoms, although some did not.

Findings from NL-SH and LASA

The analyses of the longitudinal datasets showed that hearing disability was not significantly associated with depressive symptoms. Possibly, selective losses to follow-up in both studies have diluted the effects. This means that persons with relatively more severe hearing loss (and also severe depressive symptoms) were more likely to drop out of the studies *because* of these problems. Subsequently, the perhaps already weak "real" relationship did not emerge from the data of the LASA and NL-SH participants that were still in the samples. In addition, it is known that depression has a fluctuating course, making it difficult to measure at the right moment and evidence its relationship with hearing loss (see Chapter 1).

Psychosocial health effects due to the *rate of decline* in hearing

The decline in a person's hearing ability over time was long viewed as being the mere result of a natural aging process. Nowadays, the etiology is considered more multifactorial, in that the decline is a combination of genetic, health-related, and environmental factors that have their impact across the life course (Van Eyken et al., 2007). Age-related deterioration of the ability to recognize speech in noise appears to speed up around the ages of 50 years (Stam et al., 2015) and 75 years (Pronk et al., 2013). However, these and other studies have shown that – independent of these age-differences – there are still large individual differences in each person's longitudinal pattern of decline. This also highlights why the time spent in each phase of the patient journey may vary markedly from person to person (see Chapter 13). In other words, given that the *rate* of decline differs greatly from person to person this may also affect how PHLs cope with and adapt to their hearing loss.

Up until 2013, there were no studies addressing the question of whether or not the rate of hearing loss was associated with psychosocial health. It is first important to indicate the differences between adaptation and coping. Coping concerns an active role of the individual in adjusting to changing conditions whereas adaptation also covers passive and more or less automatic processes of habituation (see Andersson et al., 1996). It can be hypothesized that when hearing declines only slowly it may require only small behavioral and emotional adjustments, whereas relatively fast declines may require more rigorous adjustments. In the former case, adaptation may play a more prominent role. In the latter case, active coping may be required more often and, generally, the chances may be larger that the overall adjustment is less successful and thus leads to more psychosocial distress during the journey of hearing loss. Further, as a slower hearing decline may go unnoticed more often, causing automatic adaptation to occur, in turn resulting in relatively less distress.

In contrast, a different perspective can be applied, yielding a different hypothesis. The concept of reduced responsiveness to chronic functional impairment assumes that in a process of increasing physical impairment, the impairment has a reduced impact on psychological outcomes over time (automatic adaptation; see Schilling et al., 2011). This occurs when reactions to an outcome variable triggered by an impaired condition attenuate in the end when the condition continues or is repeated across time. Applied to hearing loss, adaptation would work such that with continued hearing decline, further functional decline does not cause any *more* psychosocial worsening. Thus, the reduced responsiveness mechanism would cause an attenuating relationship between hearing decline and psychosocial health status across accumulated exposure to hearing problems. In line with this, the relationship between the *rate* of hearing decline and the decrease in psychosocial health would also be weaker for those with a decline from a relatively poorer baseline hearing status as they have been exposed to the hearing loss for a longer time.

Findings from NL-SH and LASA

Table 12.3 shows the longitudinal results of the studies in which the relationship between the rate of change in hearing over time (five and seven years of follow-up, respectively) and the change in social and emotional loneliness was examined. In both studies, the rate of decline in hearing was found to be associated with emotional and social loneliness. In particular, the effects applied to some subgroups only (Pronk et al., 2014; Stam et al., 2016).

Emotional and social loneliness

In the NL-SH results, particularly for non-users there was a relationship between change in hearing disability and social and emotional loneliness. Thus, feelings of social and emotional loneliness increased in participants who did not use hearing aids. Why this effect was not found in the LASA study is unknown. It could be due to the fact that determining hearing aid use is complex as report of hearing aids does not necessarily mean optimal use, or benefit from them. Further analyses of available datasets on hearing, hearing devices, and psychosocial effects are needed to provide more detailed insights into the complex relationships between these factors.

TABLE 12.3 The effects of the rate of hearing decline on social and emotional loneliness found in the Netherlands Longitudinal Study on Hearing (NL-SH) and the Longitudinal Aging Study Amsterdam (LASA)

Determinant	Outcome of interest	Sample	NL-SH	LASA
Change in hearing ability*	Change in emotional loneliness	Total sample	✓	✗
		Subgroup: Moderate hearing disability at baseline	–	✓
		Subgroup: Widow(er)s	–	✓
		Non-hearing aid users	✓	✗
	Change in social loneliness	Total sample	✓	✗
		Subgroup: Moderate hearing disability at baseline	–	✓
		Subgroup: Non-hearing aid users	✓	✗

* Measured by the digit triplet speech-in-noise test.
✓ Effect was tested and was present (statistically significant).
✗ Effect was tested and was not present (not statistically significant).
– Subgroup effect was not investigated.

Regarding the LASA findings, only significant effects for particular subgroups of older persons emerged. The strongest effect appeared for older persons who had lost their partner within the past three to four years. It may be that partner death had largely depleted the general reserves of the widow(er)s, impeding successful coping with hearing loss. Another explanation may be that persons with relatively larger hearing decline over time were restricted in seeking and finding emotional support in other, or new close ties to a greater extent than persons with smaller or no hearing decline over time. This seems in accordance with findings from a different study that used LASA data. It was found that the degree of self-reported hearing ability was not important for the continuation of existing relationships in older persons' social networks, but was important for the start of new relationships. Presumably, for the LASA respondents who recently lost their partner, their decline in hearing hampered them in making new ties or strengthening more remote ties that would have provided them again with the satisfactory deep or intimate relationship they previously had with their partner.

The second subgroup effect in LASA was found for those who deteriorated from an already moderately impaired hearing to begin with. This was in contrast to those whose hearing deteriorated from no or only mildly impaired hearing, or for those who already had a poor hearing at baseline. Taking these findings together, they suggest that in the first stage of age-related hearing loss, hearing decline does not noticeably affect social life activities, and does not affect loneliness so much. Second, in persons whose hearing deteriorates from an already moderate level of hearing loss, loneliness *is* related to the rate of hearing decline. And third, for those whose hearing is already poor, the so-called reduced responsiveness gets the upper hand, and thus the speed of further hearing deterioration does not affect loneliness.

Depression

In both NL-SH and LASA, the rate of decline in hearing was not significantly associated with depression. This may again be explained by the fluctuating course of depressive symptoms across the life span. Perhaps depressive symptoms occur only shortly after the emergence of new hearing problems, and diminish over time due to successful coping. In other words, any depressive feeling caused by hearing declines may have disappeared at the follow-up measurements.

Implications of subgroup effects for clinical and future research practice

The reported findings are relevant both for future epidemiological studies and for clinical practice. Regarding the former, the subgroup effects found for loneliness first need to be replicated in other (population-based) samples. Additionally, the underlying mechanisms that were hypothesized need to be tested in future studies to understand via which pathways hearing loss influences loneliness. Nonetheless, clinicians should be aware that loneliness risks might apply to particular subgroups of PHL. Acknowledging the preventive effects of hearing aids and the importance of monitoring the rate of hearing decline would be an adequate approach in this respect. The subgroup effects observed for partner status underline the already recognized importance in this book of involving communication partners (CPs) in the patient journey. CPs can play an important role throughout the personal and emotional stages of change the PHL goes through.

Overall, the LASA and NL-SH results suggest the importance of audiological rehabilitation through hearing aids, but additionally indicate that rehabilitation goes beyond instrumentation and should take a PHL's broader and unique context into account (e.g., gender, partner status). PHLs may require continued psychological and social support to adapt and to live with hearing loss. In this light, change in hearing and coping over time should be considered while planning management strategies to address wider consequences of hearing loss. In Chapter 2 the complex interaction between the biological, psychological, and social aspects have been highlighted. Furthermore, Chapter 13 illustrates the need for continued psychological and social support for PHLs and CPs.

Summary

Hearing disability can seriously impact PHLs' psychosocial health on their journey through hearing loss. Findings from carefully designed large epidemiological studies, and particularly prospective cohort studies, are needed to provide strong evidence for causal links between hearing disability and poor psychosocial health. Findings from two large Dutch ongoing prospective cohort studies (LASA and NL-SH) provide evidence that hearing disability causes increased feelings of social and emotional loneliness in both older and younger adults.

Not only hearing loss per se, but also the *rate* of hearing decline appears relevant: relatively faster decline causes stronger feelings of emotional and social loneliness. A key finding of LASA and NL-SH is that negative effects on loneliness seem to be particularly confined to specific subgroups of adults (e.g., men, non-hearing aid users). CPs appear to play a determining role in explaining why particular subgroups (e.g., PHL living with a partner, or PHL who recently became a widow[er]) appeared to be especially vulnerable for becoming lonely because of their hearing problems. The underlying mechanisms behind the subgroup effects are not yet fully understood and require further study.

References

Andersson, G., Melin, L., Lindberg, P., and Scott, B., 1996. Elderly hearing-impaired persons' coping behavior. *International Journal of Behavioural Medicine*, 3(4), pp. 303–320.

Bhopal, R., 2002. *Concepts of epidemiology: An integrated introduction to the ideas, theories, principles, and methods of epidemiology.* Oxford, UK: Oxford University Press.

De Jong Gierveld, J., 1998. A review of loneliness: Concept and definitions, determinants and consequences. *Review of Clinical Gerontology*, 8(1), pp. 73–80.

Garstecki, D. and Erler, S., 1999. Older adult performance on the communication profile for the hearing impaired. *Journal of Speech, Language, and Hearing Research*, 42(4), pp. 785–796.

Granberg, S., Pronk, M., Swanepoel, De W., et al., 2014. The ICF core sets for hearing loss project: Functioning and disability from the patient perspective. *International Journal of Audiology*, 53(11), pp. 777–786.

Hoogendijk, E.O., Deeg, D.J.H., Poppelaars, J., et al., 2016. The Longitudinal Aging Study Amsterdam: cohort update 2016 and major findings. *European Journal of Epidemiology*, 31, pp. 927–945.

Noble, W. and Hétu, R., 1994. An ecological approach to disability and handicap in relation to impaired hearing. *International Journal of Audiology*, 33(2), pp. 117–126.

Pronk, M., Deeg, D., Smits, C., van Tilburg, T., Kuik, D., Festen, J., and Kramer, S., 2011. Prospective effects of hearing status on loneliness and depression in older adults: Identification of subgroups. *International Journal of Audiology*, 50(12), pp. 887–896.

Pronk, M., Deeg, D., Festen, J., Twisk, J., Smits, C., Comijs, H., and Kramer, S., 2013. Decline in older persons' ability to recognize speech in noise: The influence of demographic, health-related, environmental, and cognitive factors. *Ear and Hearing*, 34(6), pp. 722–732.

Pronk, M., Deeg, D., Smits, C., Twisk, J., Festen, J., and Kramer, S., 2014. Decline in hearing ability in older persons: Does the rate of decline affect psychosocial health? *Journal of Aging Health*, 26(5), pp. 703–723.

Schilling, O. K., Wahl, H. W., Horowitz, A., Reinhardt, J. P., and Boerner, K., 2011. The adaptation dynamics of chronic functional impairment: What we can learn from older adults with vision loss. *Psychology and Aging*, 26, pp. 203–213.

Smits, C., Kapteyn, T., and Houtgast, T., 2004. Development and validation of an automatic speech-in-noise screening test by telephone. *International Journal of Audiology*, 43(1), pp. 15–28.

Stam, M., Smits, C., Twisk, J., Lemke, U., Festen, J., and Kramer, S., 2015. Deterioration of speech recognition ability over a period of 5 years in adults ages 18 to 70 years. *Ear and Hearing*, 36(3), pp. 129–137.

Stam, M., Smit, J., Twisk, J., Lemke, U., Smits, C., Festen, J., and Kramer, S., 2016. Change in psychosocial health status over five years in relation to adults' hearing ability over time. *Ear and Hearing*, in press.

Van Eyken, E., Van Camp, G., and Van Laer, L., 2007. The complexity of age-related hearing impairment: Contributing environmental and genetic factors. *Audiology and Neuro-otology*, 12(6), pp. 345–358.

World Health Organization, 2001. *International Classification of Functioning, Disability and Health (ICF)*. Geneva, Switzerland: World Health Organization.

13

EXAMPLES OF THE JOURNEY THROUGH HEARING LOSS

Ann-Christine Gullacksen

Introduction

Before we end this book in terms of the patient journey model and move on to its application, we will present the "storyline" based on one of the only long-term qualitative investigations of living with hearing loss. This chapter will provide insights into experiences of persons with hearing loss (PHLs) as a whole journey based on real narratives and examples.

At present, there is some, but not enough knowledge about how an acquired hearing loss affects personal life and what obstacles a PHL must overcome and learn to handle. Hearing problems may vary greatly depending on situations, environments, and personal factors (e.g., the person's actual state of health and mood) as described in Chapter 1. Some problems are not obviously connected to the person's hearing ability and individual reactions may be difficult to understand. In some activities, a hearing loss will have major impact on the person's engagement and have almost none in others. Both internal and external factors, and the interaction of the two, are involved and thus influence the situation. Areas critically affected may be: self-image and identity, master roles in life, relationships to significant others, work situation, and planning for future life (Engelund, 2006; Kyle et al., 1985; Manchaiah and Stephens, 2011; Gullacksen et al., 2012). Considering all this, it is important to describe these happenings from the person's point of view, from an insider perspective.

In this chapter, results will be presented from a longitudinal qualitative study of PHLs interviewed over a period of 13 years. Their narratives describe the process of learning to live with an acquired hearing loss. The seven phases of the patient journey model have been condensed into three main stages (i.e., before, during, and after rehabilitation).

Research about life change

For many years, international research has been studying psychosocial adjustment to various chronic illnesses or disabilities in a wider biopsychosocial perspective. Both empirical and theoretical knowledge have enriched our understanding of life change as a dynamic and complex process, occurring within the person. Many aspects of how life is affected in such situations have been explored in research (Chan et al., 2009).

Various models to explain life changes following disease and disability have been presented as *sequence of stages* (ibid). These stages comprise the dynamic process of adaptation, from diagnosis to the inclusion of the disability in a satisfactory life. Some stage models go beyond that and includes the time before diagnosis when insidious symptoms may affect daily life, as discussed in Chapters 3–6. This initial period can be of great emotional strain and has proven to be crucial to complete a satisfying life adjustment.

Describing the process in stages makes the person's experiences and reactions understandable to themselves, communication partners (CPs), and to the rehabilitation team. Stage of change models may give the impression that the journey through hearing loss is linear, when it is not (Smedema et al., 2009). A person may go back and forth across the phases, pause and go on later, or have a variety of events in different life domains as described in Chapter 3. Current research proves that how the journey develops depends on the person's social situation and mental conditions. All these personal matters influence how long the process will last for each individual. Individual characteristics of the process are clearly illustrated in Chapters 5–12.

Psychosocial adjustment to hearing loss

The life adjustment model describes the psychosocial adjustment as a process in three stages. *The first stage* comprises the person's early experiences before the hearing loss has been confirmed (pre-awareness, awareness, and movement phases presented in Chapter 3). The person notices vague communication problems, which increase over time causing gloomy troubles in different life areas. It is a period of growing strain and worry often long before the person seeks consultation. Eventually problems reach a *tipping point* when the person's ability to handle them has been exceeded. The hearing loss must be acknowledged as a fact and as a problem that must be faced. The tipping point triggers a transition into *the second stage* of the process. This often starts with an emotional reaction to the fact that life is about to change in a way that seems undesirable or out of control. Gradually, the PHL engages in rehabilitation and explores possible ways of handling hearing loss to reduce its negative effects. The PHL must process both personal and environmental changes. *The third stage* is a period of consolidating what has been achieved during life adjustment and rehabilitation. The themes in this process are described in the table below.

TABLE 13.1 Stages and themes in life adjustment process

Stage I: Before rehabilitation	Stage II: During rehabilitation	Stage III: After rehabilitation
• Striving back • Tipping point	• Mourning • Rehabilitation • Exploring	• Restoring • Stabilizing

Transitions between stages can be more or less obvious and some PHLs may regress or pause in their processing depending on their life situation. It is also apparent that adjustment might occur at the same time in different life domains such as family and work, each with its own agenda. Since the hearing loss can affect various life domains differently, it could take a longer or shorter time to regain control in different parts of life (see also Chapters 1 and 3). The life adjustment model is summarized in Figure 13.1.

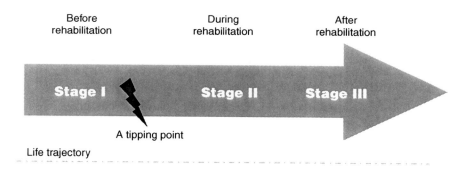

FIGURE 13.1 Life adjustment model

The longitudinal study

In this chapter, results are presented from a longitudinal qualitative study about psychosocial adjustment in the case of hearing loss. This study appears to be the longest following of PHLs to explore the consequences of hearing loss.

This research is comprised of three sub-studies performed in Sweden during a period of 13 years, 1990–2003. In the first study, 33 PHLs were interviewed (aged 27 to 63). In the second study, 25 of them were interviewed again and in the last study, 19 remained to be interviewed. Across the whole study, a total of 85 interviews were conducted. All participants had confirmed hearing loss; some had used a hearing aid for many years, others for just a few months. Some had had a hearing loss since childhood, identified then or later in life. Most of them had experienced a gradual hearing loss in adulthood. Furthermore, many of them had some kind of ear disease and tinnitus.

The life adjustment process used to analyze the interviews has been developed in a study about women learning to live with chronic pain (Gullacksen and Lidbeck, 2004). The life adjustment model has since been tested both in research focusing on various diagnoses and in clinical rehabilitation practice. An overall biopsychosocial perspective on life transition shapes the theoretical framework as presented in Chapters 1 and 2.

The first stage (before): striving back and tipping point

Some of the participants in this study were just beginning to recognize their hearing problems, sometimes very reluctantly. Some had already started their rehabilitation and were testing a hearing aid. All of them could tell a unique and personal story of their experiences during this initial stage.

In 1990, during the first interviews, some interesting points were made that became important concepts and phenomena to further explore in the interviews following. The most interesting was the very distinct *tipping point* that made the person ready to face life changes. This phenomenon in this early stage was more or less obvious in all stories. It could be identified sometimes as very strong reactions and fatigue, sometimes more moderate and controllable. The participants often describe the time before the tipping point as "going down a slope until you hit the ground." They felt overloaded with stress, denied or concealed problems that occur increasingly frequently, and were gradually losing control over daily situations. All this more or less affected their self-concept and self-confidence. The fact that their problems reached beyond the actual hearing loss was for some at first incomprehensible. Emerging problems were noticed in job situations, relations, performance, and overall social life.

During the early part of this stage, several of the participants recall a strong *urge to go back* to the well-known life course in which they were invested. The person struggled to go back to what still was considered to be one's "normal life," safe and under control. This often was furthered by a strong drive and motivation to hold on to the past and reject the unknown intruder in life. Situations that used to be predictable and taken for granted (e.g., meeting people, conversations, getting information), are recognized as being no longer reliable. The desire to resume activities, work, important social roles and so on was strengthened by a drive to hold onto self-esteem and self-identity. It became a fight to find coping strategies to handle daily life in socially accepted ways. Gradually their self-identity fell into question because they did not know if they had heard correctly and reacted as expected. At this point, uncertainty comes creeping into fundamental feelings of safety and control that so far had kept life together.

An important observation from the interviews was the participants' strategic work to keep up their personal and expected image; it was kept *behind the scenes, out of sight of others*. Such efforts could include: selecting and disclosing strategies which reduce embarrassing situations; living up to expectations and self-image; checking information and so on. These efforts increased the workload for PHLs and as a consequence resulted in restricted ability to concentrate on other life events. The concept of *behind the scenes* demonstrates how the person builds an overload of strain not seen by others until a breakthrough, when the curtain falls and reveals the situation. Such situations were frequently reported, mostly from the working life.

Let's consider some case examples:

David struggled with emerging hearing problems at work as a sales manager. He experienced daily stresses to his performances at work. When he went to work in the morning, he worried about what hassles he would be forced to tackle during the day. The staff leader was surprised when David told him that he could not manage his work situation any more, and said, "None of us have suspected that you have such hearing problems. You should have told us long before. We could have helped you." David recalls later that he, at the time, couldn't put words to his problems and talk about them. He also carefully considered what it could mean to his position at the company if he revealed his problems.

Many of the interviewees remember that they felt very lonely during this time. They had difficulties in understanding or finding words to talk about their feelings and experiences to others (see Chapters 5 and 6 on pre-awareness and awareness phases).

Often family members will be the first to notice the hearing problems. During the time before the tipping point, there will continuously be situations of irritation and strain in family relations. Some of the participants also noticed that family members really did not have any idea about all the work behind the scenes that was part of the PHL's daily life.

The interviews revealed that the motivation for "striving back" fades while the personal experiences of daily problems increase and become a burden they cannot handle. The tipping point implies that the person's motivation may shift direction from striving back to prepare for changes in present life.

When reaching the tipping point, many of the participants discuss ill health, stress symptoms or stress-induced illness, burn-out symptoms, and exhaustion. They gave all their strength during work hours and had to withdraw and rest at home. Some remember that they reached a point when a weekend was not enough to be fit to go back to work. They felt they had come to a dead-end and said, "You have to stop!" Several of the participants had to take sick leave for a while before they could consider what to do about their lives.

Triggers for change

Many of the interviewees recalled the tipping point as triggered by a very distinct experience. Such triggers could be quite trivial episodes, but resulted in a dramatic change for the person.

Betty told how impressed she was when she saw one of the directors at the firm using a hearing aid. She thought: "If he can, I can."

Anna was not ready to contact the hearing clinic until one day at the lunch restaurant she observed a woman wearing a hearing aid quite visibly. Anna remembers this incident very clearly. Her immediate thought was, "She looks quite normal!" This reflection affected her a lot and confronted her with the fear of being stigmatized by others who discovered her hearing problems. Instead of neglecting problems, she felt ready to do something about them. She thought this very sudden decision was a result of an unconscious preparation in her mind that had been going on for some time.

Karen had for some years resisted the family's attempts to get her to contact the hearing clinic. She recalls with a smile how her daughter changed this. The six-year-old daughter saw a man at the bus wearing a hearing aid and said: "Why don't you get one of those 'talking-machines' to your ear?" This became Karen's trigger to change.

For **Dorothy**, it was an embarrassing situation at work. She recalls that she for many months struggled to manage her work as a nurse assistant while her hearing problems worsened. One day at the morning meeting, she lost track of what was said and suddenly she heard the group leader say: "Dorothy, you take responsibility for this matter and report back." She had no idea what was expected of her and panicked. She then understood that she could not continue like this and had to do something about it.

For others the trigger could be connected to acute health problems stemming from living with strain in life for a long time, or to family matters, as, "I really like to hear the voices of my grandchildren."

The significance of the tipping point

The participants' shift in attitude towards their increasing problems in hearing situations proved to be crucial for a successful adjustment process. The tipping point emerged when the person admitted that the hearing loss was the cause of his or her problems combined with the feeling of doing something about it. This changeover could be found in all stories, often very distinct and for some more vague. It was obvious that realizing facts about one's hearing ability is not the same as realizing and understanding its consequences in life. This acknowledgment can be described as comprehending on a cognitive level (Chan et al., 2009). It was obvious though, that realizing facts is a crucial and vital first step to take an active part in processing what the hearing loss means in life.

This new perspective on problems often led the person to seek help at a hearing clinic. The participants described this as a quite new confrontation to their problems. Fitting a hearing aid usually is a consultation over time, which means that it will continue along the person's ongoing overall life adjustment process in the second stage.

Summary: the first stage before rehabilitation

Significant for this first stage of adjustment is that it can occur for long periods of time, sometimes for years. The emerging consequences in life are not immediately identified as caused by a hearing problem. The person struggles to keep up with duties and expectations in life and conceals difficulties and strain. For some it is hard to put words to worries and thoughts, which delays consultation. The result is a feeling of being alone with growing concerns. For many the tipping point marks the beginning of emotional and social adjustment to include the hearing loss in life. For some the tipping point later in the rehabilitation was disclosed as a sign of striving back to the well-known life and not driven by a motivation to change in life (see Betty's example below). Hence, it is important to recognize these persons early in the rehabilitation and support them (see Chapter 6).

Not all PHLs have experienced a long and trying start to the life adjustment process. Even so, many of them recall these types of emotions, but may not describe them in terms of crises, depression, or panic. However, it is important to identify those who give signs of having difficulties in the shift of attitude towards the impairment.

The second stage (during): mourning and exploring

The transition from the tipping point to the second stage in the adjustment process was more or less obvious in the participants' stories. The beginning of this stage is characterized by a period of despair, sadness, and for some, a fearful loss of control over the life course. For many of them the tipping point released their long suppressed feelings about what a hearing loss might mean to them. The life they were settled in and had invested in until now seemed lost and unreachable. At the same time, they felt both defeat and relief when their problems became recognized.

A leading theme throughout this stage is restoration of self-esteem, self-identity, and self-confidence that have been exposed to severe doubts during the first stage. Some participants described that they felt that their identity was taken over by the hearing disability.

Emmy struggled to find herself in the image she thought others had of her now: "Here comes Emmy with a hearing loss!" The mission was to find her way back to the "true me" and at the same time include the hearing loss as one of many parts of the person she wanted to be. For some this was an exhausting and emotional struggle.

Karen told that by discovering the person she really was and had suppressed, she became eager to reclaim her self-identity. She described this "as bursting out of a cocoon that had restricted my life for many years." This gave her possibilities to try new activities and enlarge her social life. This was a happy shift for Karen but in the beginning confused both family and friends who had to adjust their view of her. Not all of the participants could discover a desirable and forgotten identity like Karen. Some had to reconstruct a new one that gradually could include the hearing loss and give satisfaction.

During this fragile time, a PHL is also occupied with hearing rehabilitation. Some of the interviewees recalled how they were flung between hope and despair. In many ways, the hearing aid facilitated everyday life, but it also aroused an emotional strain connected to the personal identity of having a hearing loss.

Most participants had invested great hope in the hearing aid and expected it to eliminate all their hearing problems. Nevertheless, they were often unprepared to meet with new and unexpected problems connected to making use of the hearing aid. For some the rehabilitation confronted them with the full range of consequences in life caused by the hearing loss, which came as a shock and changed hope into disappointment. Some interviews indicate that it could take years before the person went back to the hearing clinic to seek help a second time.

Betty's story below illustrates such a situation. In five years, she had endured a troublesome life change that had not yet come to a satisfactory ending. She struggled to hold on to her personal identity strongly connected to her lifestyle. Betty was interviewed on two occasions in 1990 and 1995.

Betty had had different jobs earlier, and now worked at an office where she had daily contact with customers. Her problems had become increasingly exhausting and her friends took her to the hearing clinic. When she was first interviewed, she just had her first hearing aid. She emphasized that she "really was not a hearing impaired person" although she could have problems now and then. Her story gave examples of daily stress situations both at work and in her spare time. When I met her five years later, she was on sick leave due to several health problems triggered by overwhelming stress. She had not used her hearing aids during these years because she could not adjust to them and felt they were negative in general. She had not turned to the hearing clinic to discuss these problems further and had had no follow-up from the clinic. Now she was in contact with a rehabilitation team at her workplace and they had told her to start using her hearing aids. She was devastated. Her earlier lifestyle was full of activities and challenges in working life and in social life. But, not anymore. The hearing loss hindered her from keeping up her desired lifestyle. She still fights the fact of the hearing loss. Her personal adjustment process has not been successful. She still struggles to find a way to adjust her life.

For most participants, emotional reactions faded and the motivation to explore life and different environments grew stronger. The fitting of a hearing aid gave reason to explore oneself in different settings with or without the hearing aid. Exploring involves trying out proper hearing strategies and coping strategies that could be reliable to further regain control over performance in daily life. The participants' stories reveal that there is an ongoing inner dialog to consider different ways to perform, handle, and confront everyday situations. All this exploring has to be done together with the efforts to strengthen the self and personal identity in various settings. Therefore, engaging in hearing rehabilitation must be seen as a parallel process to life adjustment, both strongly connected and influencing each other. As Martin says below, it is also a learning process.

Martin concludes, "You have to face all kinds of situations to learn to estimate options, hindrance, personal involvement, the meaning of the situation and so on. You have to find courage to go on, not only strength."

Summary: the second stage during rehabilitation

The second stage often starts with the feeling of having lost the future and at the same time having nothing to return to. However, as the examples illustrate this stage could end in a more hopeful mode. For most PHLs, it will be a period of going through rehabilitation – technical as well as at work. At the same time, the PHLs are also experiencing several personal adjustments to cope with the consequences of hearing loss; often these adjustments are going on "behind the scenes." These personal efforts to restore life have proved to be important to a successful rehabilitation.

The third stage (after): rebuilding, restoring, and stabilizing

The transition to the third stage in the life adjustment process is not as distinctive as between the first and second. Yet, there is a clear difference to be found in the personal attitude towards the hearing loss. The participants became more purposeful in their seeking of solutions and less generally exploring. They were aware of the demands derived from the hearing loss, but also aware of how far they themselves wanted to compromise about role-performance in different contexts. They had learned to estimate the costs they invested and value the benefits they gained in various situations and engagements.

Coming this far in the process, the PHLs were better prepared to act assertively: to tackle circumstances in their environments, to explain the hearing situation to others, and to demand adjustments needed (see Chapter 12). They experienced less daily strain. It was obvious that the PHLs had regained control over life. They grew increasingly skillful at handling new situations and relations. They had found a likeable self-identity and experienced a satisfying quality of life including the hearing loss.

By now, family members had learned to understand what the hearing loss meant in daily life and had time to find their own strategies to cope. Family and close friends had developed supportive strategies that could prevent problems emerging in social life. Some participants had chosen to live alone since this gave them full control over planning their life in a suitable way considering their hearing problems.

Summary: the third stage after rehabilitation

At this stage, the person's control over how to handle the hearing loss increases. Daily life is restored and life satisfaction is accessible. Nevertheless, relapses to the second stage could occur, although this does not warrant additional technical rehabilitation. However, these PHLs might need other kinds of support in terms of psychological and social support, which then are often missed at the clinic. The main component in the third stage is to make the PHLs feel confident to handle any unexpected and challenging hearing situations.

Maintenance work

Already in the first interviews, it became obvious that having passed a successful life adjustment process did not mean that the hearing problems were solved forever. It was very clear in this longitudinal study that the PHLs continued strategic work to facilitate life with hearing loss. They had constant maintenance work to do.

All participants described that they always had a watchful eye in social situations. This monitoring was a way to keep control over life and it gave a feeling of mastery. They assessed which coping strategies could be required, what was at stake in a situation, and calculated costs and benefits in encounters. This extra work was mentioned as an accustomed behavior in daily life. It was not exposed to others and was carefully concealed. This illustrates that *the work behind the scenes* continues as a part of the PHL's daily life. This extra work still costs energy and a main task was to reduce their mental effort.

Margaret said: "I am used to this way of living. I have a habit of always listening. I can't relax as I think a hearing person can. Nevertheless, I can't say I have any daily problems anymore."

The maintenance work could increase in periods (e.g., caused by a temporary ear infection, tinnitus, or by external factors like a reorganization at work, social disturbances in life and so on). In such situations, sudden occurrence of hearing problems surprised others and gave rise to misunderstandings. The PHLs strived to avoid such situations and therefore tried very hard not to disclose their maintenance work. However, they had learned not to worry ahead. "You can't worry over things that might come" was a frequent conclusion.

From the PHLs' stories, it is clear that they very often use the same strategies to reduce stress in everyday situations as in the first stage of the adjustment process. The difference is that now these are carefully valued and chosen to give the best possible benefit in the situation.

Comments on rehabilitation

Many stories reveal the tribulation that PHLs go through before seeking consultation. This also indicates that enabling early rehabilitation requires a program that can identify these persons' needs when they first visit the clinic. Interviews in this study show that people sometimes contacted the hearing clinic during the period of vague hearing problems but were not offered further rehabilitation or follow-up. Betty's story above is an example of this kind. She started to be fitted with a hearing aid, but disappointedly ended the rehabilitation and was not given any follow-up.

Most crucial in the rehabilitation process is *to give the right support* or proposal *at the most suited time* for the individual. This timing requires qualified professional knowledge and experience. Models proposed in this book can be of great help. The life adjustment model can be a guide to understand the person's whole life situation, including the meaning of the hearing loss. The PHL must be the leading person in the rehabilitation process since this also involves their personal work of adjustment behind the scenes, as described in the second stage above. This underlines the importance of letting the person be in control of the planning, timing, and pace of the rehabilitation process.

The participants in the study described what kind of support they preferred during the adjustment process. The overall most important support was an understanding attitude from family and close friends. Next to this came support from professionals who gave them facts and information to understand their condition. This also helped to explain to others their situation. Hence, there is a clear need to involve CPs in the audiological rehabilitation sessions (Manchaiah et al., 2012). Many also mentioned contact with other PHLs as a special and comforting support.

Summary

It has been argued throughout this book that there is a need for adopting a person-centered audiological rehabilitation (PCAR). PCAR primarily focuses on the hearing loss and a well-fitted hearing aid. Nevertheless, it is a well-known fact that a hearing loss is associated with a large range of personal consequences in physical, mental, and social life domains as discussed in Chapter 1. A correctly fitted hearing aid surely improves hearing function but many problems connected to the hearing disability will remain. It is important that the practitioner has a sense for signs that might indicate a hidden agenda deriving from psychosocial issues in the person's life. Several studies conclude that a holistic approach in rehabilitation is needed to understand the person's awareness process and readiness to confront the problems.

The longitudinal study discussed in this chapter confirms that going through a life adjustment process is a major life event and for most people is long-term hard work. Hence, this clearly demonstrates that the PCAR should be much more than instrumentation (e.g., hearing aids) and there is a great need for providing psychosocial support to help PHLs continue to adapt and live with hearing loss.

References

Chan, F., Da Silva Cardoso, E., and Chronister, J. (Eds.), 2009. *Understanding Psychosocial Adjustment to Chronic Illness and Disability: A Handbook for Evidence-Based Practitioners in Rehabilitation.* New York, NY: Springer Publishing Company.

Engelund, G., 2006. *Time for hearing – recognising process for the individual – a grounded theory.* Unpublished doctoral thesis. Department of Nordic Studies and Linguistics Audiologopedics. Eriksholm, Denmark: University of Copenhagen, and Oticon Research Centre.

Gullacksen, A.-C. and Lidbeck, J., 2004. The life adjustment process in chronic pain: Psychosocial assessment and clinical implications. *Pain Research Management,* 9(3), pp. 145–153.

Gullacksen, A.-C., Göransson, L., Henningsen Rönnblom, G., Koppen, A., and Rud Jörgensen, A., 2012. Life adjustment and combined visual and hearing disability/deafblindness – An internal process over time. *Nordic Welfare Centre* [online]. Available at: www.nordicwelfare. org/Publications/Livsomstallning/ [Accessed on 16 March 2016].

Kyle, J., Jones, L., and Wood, P., 1985. Adjustment to acquired hearing loss: A working model. In H. Orlans (Ed.), *Adjustment to Adult Hearing Loss.* London, UK: Taylor & Francis.

Manchaiah, V. and Stephens, D., 2011. The patient journey: Living with hearing impairment. *Journal of the Academy of Rehabilitative Audiology,* 44, pp. 29–40.

Manchaiah, V., Stephens, D., Zhao, F., and Kramer, S., 2012. The role of communication partners in the audiological enablement/rehabilitation of a person with hearing impairment: An overview. *Audiological Medicine*, 10(1), pp. 21–30.

Smedema, A., Bakken-Gillen, S., and Dalton, J., 2009. Psychosocial adaptation to chronic illness and disability: Models and measurement. In F. Chan, E. Da Silva Cardoso, and J. Chronister (Eds.), *Understanding Psychosocial Adjustment to Chronic Illness and Disability: A Handbook for Evidence-Based Practitioners in Rehabilitation*. New York, NY: Springer Publishing Company.

14

PRACTICE IMPLICATIONS OF THE PATIENT JOURNEY MODEL

Hans Henrik Philipsen and Melanie Gregory

Introduction

The patients benefit immensely from understanding their hearing loss as a journey through different phases with diverse challenges and needs. This more holistic approach creates an understanding and insight to what and why hearing loss and its consequences are happening and hence to what can be done. The patients' insight gained from understanding their own journey and that they are not alone fosters a stronger engagement, motivation, and hence self-management to take action on the hearing loss. This is realized through feedback often received from clinics: "the patients are better equipped to make decisions that are right for them and to guide us on the support they need throughout their hearing journey."

The possible patient journey

The Ida Institute's own journey to creation of the patient journey model is closely related to a person-centered outlook on the world of hearing loss. The aim of the institute was to develop a tool for hearing care professionals that could be used as a starting point for understanding the complex phases and numerous milestones of hearing loss. This understanding would enable hearing care professionals to better address the entire patient experience and collaborate with patients to achieve better outcomes. The tool is based on the innovation of 65 prominent and distinguished international hearing care professionals participating in a series of innovation seminars. This possible patient journey model has six phases (see Figure 14.1), which include: (1) Pre-awareness, (2) awareness, (3) Movement, (4) Diagnostics, (5) Rehabilitation, and (6) Post-clinical. However, Manchaiah et al. (2011) have further developed the patient journey model by taking the patient's view into account (see Chapter 3).

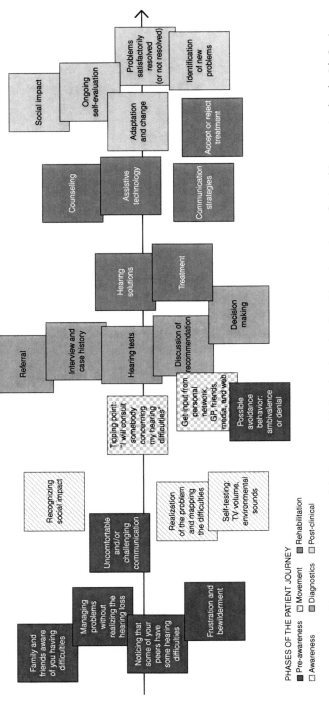

FIGURE 14.1 Possible patient journey model of person with hearing loss developed based on the professionals' perspective by the Ida Institute

PHASES OF THE PATIENT JOURNEY
■ Pre-awareness ☐ Movement ■ Rehabilitation
☐ Awareness ■ Diagnostics ☐ Post-clinical

The strength of the patient journey model is the imminent shift from the traditional vertical focus in the middle of the journey at the diagnostics phase when the clinical appointment occurs, toward the journey as a whole, starting even before people know they have a hearing problem and continuing throughout the patient's lifetime. The person-centered care that this model provides helps patients to come away with a positive experience, because their individual concerns and journey are considered. Communicating an understanding of the patients' hearing challenges and their emotional impact allows the patient to feel validated and understood, creating a foundation for a trusting therapeutic alliance (Silvester et al., 2007; Switankowsky, 2004).

As with all models that attempt to explain a complex reality simply, this model cannot fully depict all of the complexities of a patient's journey of hearing loss. However, it can be used to foster communication between patient and clinician that may challenge, re-model, or re-configure the experiences depicted, resulting in greater understanding of the human dynamics of hearing loss. It is a way to establish a shared understanding of the patient experience, which is a necessary starting point for decision making and action.

By the time a patient comes to see hearing healthcare professionals, the patient has usually experienced several different phases. Many of those stages are recognizable but patients also bring unique characteristics of their journey with them. In recognition of each individual's unique experience of hearing loss, the patient journey tool uses broad phrases and suggests experiences typical of each phase to enhance practitioner and patient understanding of the broader context of hearing loss (see Table 14.1).

Changing behavior

Before consensus was reached on the linear model of the possible patient journey model, several Ida seminar participants drew iterative circles to indicate that people with hearing loss often go through re-fitting processes and hit-the-wall relapses that necessitate a return to a previous phase.

The Ida Institute followed up on this approach with the circular model, a cyclical representation of the stages of change that a person with hearing loss (PHL) may confront when considering aspects of audiological rehabilitation (Prochaska and Di Clemente, 1984). The circular model is based on the different phases and processes a PHL experiences when changing behavior (see Figure 14.2).

The circular model provides a visual representation of patients' state of mind during different phases of their rehabilitation, as well as the types of clinician interactions that may foster change. Self-assessment from the patient combined with the clinician's observations help to focus the discussion around the patient's readiness for change.

The circular model is used to track present and future motivational levels of the patient with regards to behavior change. It also provides guidance for the hearing care professional on communication tactics to support the changing process at each specific stage in the most efficient way. Most patients will experience the changing process several times before the new behavior is well established and integrated.

TABLE 14.1 Recommendations for hearing healthcare professionals using the patient journey model to foster person-centered care

Phase in the patient journey model	What to do?
Pre-awareness: The patient is experiencing communication problems but may be managing without acknowledging the hearing problem. The patient may feel bewildered or frustrated. Family and friends may begin to notice the patient's hearing difficulties.	Engage in activities that raise awareness of the hearing problem. Encourage the patient to keep a diary of times when communication is challenging. Support the patient in identifying situations that are affected by hearing. Listen to the patient and provide clear, short, and specific information.
Awareness: The patient realizes that hearing loss is impacting his or her social and work life. The patient may recognize hearing loss and begin to map the problems it causes. The patient may "self-test" by raising the TV volume or by attempting to control other environmental sounds.	Listen to the patient. Explore their experiences with hearing and communication. Explore ambivalence about hearing help-seeking. Provide brief advice about hearing and communication options.
Movement: The patient reaches a "tipping point" and is ready to consult with a hearing care professional. The patient gathers information about hearing loss from a variety of sources, including his or her personal network, general practitioner, media, and the internet.	Focus on the benefits of hearing. Provide options and choices. Provide relevant information specific to the patient's daily life needs regarding hearing and communication.
Diagnostics: The patient actively seeks referral to a hearing care professional. The patient meets with a clinician for an interview and case history, hearing test, and recommendations, leading to decision making.	Directly address patient concerns. Provide choice for hearing and communication challenges. Focus on the impact and benefit of each option on the daily life of the patient.
Rehabilitation: The patient takes action by seeking counseling, treatment, and hearing technologies (e.g., hearing aids and assistive devices). In this context, the patient develops new communication strategies and may accept or reject the recommendations of the hearing care professional.	Listen to the patient. Focus on the benefits to themselves, family, and other communication partners of improved hearing.
Self-evaluation: This new phase was identified by patients (Manchaiah, 2013) and is characterized by self-assigned reasons for their hearing loss, quantifying problems, and reflecting on the negative and positive aspects of trying hearing aids and evaluating treatment received.	Listen to the patient. Ensure that you identify what is going well and reinforce these activities. Continue to acknowledge ambivalence. Continue to set joint goals and agree specific activities that can support achievement of goals. Check that the patient has a clear understanding of the hearing problem and its implications, so that they can explain to others. Ensure that the patient can self-advocate.
Resolution: The patient undergoes adaptation to change, considers the social impact of change and the extent to which problems have been resolved.	Encourage active self-management of the hearing problem.

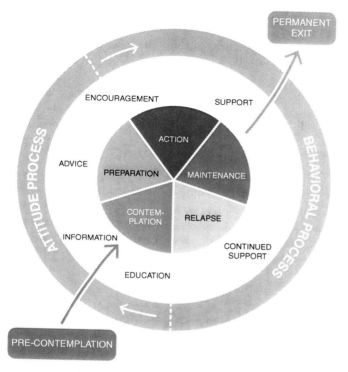

FIGURE 14.2 Circular representation of the stages of change model (adapted from Prochaska and Di Clemente, 1984)

Person-centered care beyond the clinic

In developing the possible patient journey model with seminar participants, there emerged a natural focus on the middle of the journey at the point where the hearing care professional encounters the patient. To support the paradigm shift from a focus on a techno-centric approach to a more person-centered, holistic approach, the Ida Institute explored strategies for expanding the focus to also encompass the beginning and end of the patient journey (Hickson, 2012).

The reason for this paradigm shift centers on increased patient engagement and motivation to improve hearing and communication found in PHLs who are aware of their communication needs and have already addressed some of those concerns before coming to their initial or first follow-up appointment. They are likely to be better equipped to make decisions that are right for them and to guide the hearing care professional on the support they need throughout their hearing journey. This will encourage a greater involvement in the process and assertiveness to take action and self-manage during later phases of their journey.

The role of the audiologist is not going away, but it is changing and expanding in new ways. It will require a greater flexibility, including use of tele-health, a willingness to utilize new technologies in and out of the session to aid patients, and of course, listening closely to patients' needs and wants. The counseling already occurring during appointments is going to become increasingly central to the appointment, and will require extending beyond the appointment to tailor an effective treatment plan for patients. Tele-health offers hearing care professionals an opportunity to offer individualized care beyond the physical encounter in the clinic. It calls for reframing toward a more holistic approach that fosters trust and helps to build life-long relationships with patients. Incorporating strategies to encourage shared decision making allows patients to take ownership of their hearing health and make a stronger commitment to treatment.

Tele-health can be used in different ways throughout the patient journey. It can provide information for those who are beginning to wonder if they might have a hearing loss, as well as offer resources and support for people with hearing loss and their communication partners (CPs). It enables clinicians to maintain a dialogue with patients, even if they cannot make it to the office. Thereby making hearing care increasingly accessible to a broader patient base.

Ida tele-care

The Ida Institute, working in collaboration with more than 100 internationally renowned hearing care professionals, has developed a suite of easy-to-use online tools and resources to help people with hearing loss prepare for appointments and successfully manage everyday communication and important decisions related to hearing. The online platform supports hearing care professionals in extending person-centered care beyond the clinic, creating multiple opportunities for hearing care professionals to individualize care pre- and post-appointments and build relationships and trust that enhance the therapeutic process long term.

The new online platform addresses the three main stages of the patient's journey: preparation for first appointment; preparation for follow-up appointments; and everyday life with hearing loss. Hearing care professionals can direct patients to website links with the appropriate tool or phase by email confirming appointments or even as a follow-up service to encourage patients to explore the platform resources on their own. Within each phase, there are online tools that patients can use to prepare for appointments or use as they learn to live well with their hearing loss.

These preparations support the patient in making the right decisions and guide their hearing care professional on the support they need. By encouraging patients to think about their needs and concerns ahead of time, clinicians can save time during the appointment, have more productive conversations, and develop long-term relationships. Further information can be accessed from: http://idainstitute.com/toolbox/telecare/

Mentoring through the patient journey

As demonstrated by the research and innovative tools outlined above, qualified, trustworthy, and wise guidance is critical to a successful patient journey. The *rite of passage*, a notion originally described by ethnography, has lately been reintroduced as a useful concept in healthcare to empower healthcare professionals to counsel patients successfully through difficult stages of life, e.g., treatment of cancer patients and social rehabilitation of disabled people (Waller and Sibbett, 2008; Willett and Deegan, 2001).

A successfully performed rite of passage brings order to the chaotic and confusing stages in life for those involved and for the surrounding society. It helps people understand, accept, and adapt to the necessary transitions encountered at different life stages.

In this ethnographic approach to patient care, hearing care professionals are among the experienced mentors that guide and support patients to manage their hearing loss and empower them to take action. Person-centered care (PCC) calls for strong mentors who can connect the elements of a hearing loss in a logical and meaningful way that makes the passages of the journey of hearing loss safe and understandable for patients.

The common characteristic of rites of passage is their three-way structure. First, there is the separation or detachment, second, a liminal stage, and third, a reintegration. For people experiencing hearing loss, *the separation stage* is a feeling of detachment from participating in typical social interaction with family members, at work, or even perhaps with health professionals. PHLs find their status questioned by others, as they are no longer as they "used to be." Their role as an equal conversation partner is compromised, since they are no longer capable of prompt responses in smooth conversational exchanges. An increasing detachment from normal social activity (i.e., how it was before hearing loss) is a very common form of patient feedback. A sense of belonging to "another world" is well documented.

As the hearing loss worsens, the second stage, known as *the liminal stage*, begins. In ethnographic literature and in cancer and disability studies, this stage refers to a limited period when people are between statuses and ambiguous with respect to their social identity. Admitted to a hospital, you are no longer Mr. Smith the carpenter, or Ms. Bernstein the professor. You are a patient undergoing a treatment.

The *liminal stage* is often painful for PHLs. In interviews, people report that, "you still feel that you are yourself, but you cannot be yourself, because people see you as that other person with a hearing loss" (Ida Institute, 2010). Some degree of depression often occurs in this phase on the journey. There is a sense of withdrawal from society without knowing if it is the hearing loss or perhaps dementia. Interactions with other people often become less frequent, as one avoids unnecessary social contact. The lack of hearing makes the PHL unable to conform to cross-culturally defined norms of good behavior, such as interrupting conversations, avoiding small talk, looking unengaged and uninterested, or looking "stupid" or "slow" (see Chapter 11). This can create social pain that isolates the PHL even more (MacDonald and Jensen-Campbell, 2011).

The third stage of the rite of passage is the *rite of reintegration* or "rite of rehabilitation," during which the individual returns to society with a new status.

The culmination of the reintegration into normal society almost always includes a new position, identity, and set of responsibilities. A person becomes socially visible again.

Many PHLs who have gone through hearing rehabilitation (e.g., users of hearing aids or cochlear implants) explain that getting back to an active social life is like "getting the old-new life back again" (Ida Institute, 2010). The hearing instruments, if visible at all, are a sign of people who have taken action on their hearing loss, much like the red dot (bindi) used in Southeast Asia signals that a woman has reentered society as a married woman. The changes form a part of a new identity as a hearing aid user. As is the case with any new identity or role, a responsibility and new sets of behaviors are included. For people with hearing aids, this means implementing newly adopted communication strategies to facilitate and make communication easier.

The mentoring role is crucial in this reintegration process. To get safely through obstacles on their journey, patients need guidance from dedicated hearing care providers. These experienced mentors guide and support patients through these obstacles and help them understand what to expect as they continue on their journey to living well with hearing loss.

Examples of the use of journey model by hearing healthcare professionals

Since its launch in 2009, the Ida Institute's patient journey model has been used in different settings by many hearing care professionals. Some of these professionals shared their experiences below.

Michelle Arnold, University of South Florida, United States of America

As a clinical audiology instructor, I am frequently in need of active, "hands-on" activities to bridge the gaps between theories taught in the classroom and how to apply those to patients encountered in the clinic. To expect an inexperienced clinician to understand the nuances of how a patient's life experiences impact his or her decision to seek or not seek intervention for hearing loss is unfair and, in some cases, sets both the student and the patient up for failure. I've had success using the Patient Journey as a practical approach for demonstrating how the transtheoretical model of behavior change can be applied to most patients seen in an audiology clinic at almost any point along the disease path (i.e., at any "stage" of the patient journey and experience with hearing loss). I utilize the online format of the patient journey tool, accessed from the Ida Institute website. In the classroom setting, I solicit clinical examples from doctor of audiology students based on their first experiences working in a university-based clinic. We then, as a group, begin to discuss the patient's background and history, including the reasons s/he is seeking out an audiologist to begin with. The students are responsible for determining where the knowledge, attitudes, and behaviors exhibited by the patient lie along the continuum of change. During this process, we draft the patient journey on sticky notes that are posted and rearranged as new thoughts and ideas about the patient's journey come up. Finally, we decide on a patient journey that aligns with the model of behavior change and use the online tool for a version that can be shown on a large screen. I leave the journey up during the remainder of the class and refer to it at different times throughout the lecture, relating all of the concepts and ideas back to the true expert for their own hearing loss – the patient. By allowing the students to think through a real-life example of the patient journey in the classroom, it gives them a more concrete way of considering individual differences and how they might affect outcomes. I believe that encouraging students to think of things from a patient's perspective helps eliminate the urge to "fix" problems that might not be a priority for some individuals. Further, it helps students see that perhaps there are problems that are in greater need of "fixing" that wouldn't have been considered if the patient were looked at simply in terms of their hearing status, and not as a whole.

Cherilee Rutherford, University of Cape Town, South Africa

I have used the patient journey tool in our Introduction to Amplification class at University College London, to help students think specifically about what happens in the different appointments of a hearing aid fitting journey. We set up three groups with sticky notes and divided the groups to each think about a different appointment (e.g., Assessment/HA candidacy, fitting, follow-up). Each group brainstormed all the different things that could/should happen in these various sessions and noted these on sticky notes. They then moved as a group to the next appointment type, reviewed what a previous group have done and added to that. This process is continued until all groups have had a chance to think about and contribute to each appointment. This created some lively debate and healthy competition to see if anyone left out something important! It was also an opportunity for experienced students to share their knowledge and engage in peer tutoring. The classroom was wallpapered with sticky notes but it was colorful, fun, and interactive! When one sees the sheer volume of things that go into this part of the patient journey alone, you appreciate the complexity of this process and how skilled you need to be as a professional to effectively manage all of this without dropping the ball and while maintaining a patient-centered approach to hearing care. I am keen to try this exercise again with e-tools such as Padlet (www.padlet.com).

Vinaya Manchaiah, Lamar University, Texas, United States of America

I came across the possible patient journey model that Ida Institute developed during 2009 when I attended the Ida Institute seminar in Denmark. At that point of time these were new ideas in the area of rehabilitation audiology. However, as the information presented in the model was institutive to experienced audiologists, it was the first time I considered the experiences of PHLs as a whole from the point of noticing hearing difficulties till they continue to adjust in life with hearing challenges even after audiological rehabilitation.

I have used the patient journey model mainly in three ways since then. Firstly, I used this tool in teaching undergraduate students in audiology about the experiences PHLs may have. I found this to be a very useful tool that is very helpful while explaining about the wider (individual, psychological, and social) consequences of hearing loss. Secondly, I have used this model extensively in research. The principle behind the patient journey (i.e., process evaluation) formed the main area of research during my doctoral studies. This idea in addition to the health behavior change stages-of-change models helped studying the lived experiences of PHLs in the form of a timeline. Lastly but importantly, I have used this model while addressing the hard of hearing support group in South Wales. This group consisted of adult PHLs of varying degrees and at varied stages in their journey (e.g., some successfully adopted rehabilitation whereas others just started to notice hearing difficulties). This model was presented to the members and engaging the members resulted in extensive discussions about this tool/model. In general, the PHLs were re-assured that their journey was typical as presented in the model and an accurate representation of what may happen in general. Overall, I found this model/tool to have many practical applications and only our imagination can help foster its applications.

Summary

The concept of the patient journey creates a framework that enables hearing care professionals to better understand the complexities and unique perspectives that shape each individual's experience of hearing loss. Understanding patient stories (i.e., their personal conceptualization of the history, the cause, the onset, development, and consequences of their hearing loss) is a critical starting point and a cornerstone. This understanding, reflected back to the patients, enhances their own understanding of their hearing loss and generates confidence in their ability to self-manage their hearing loss. Although hearing is a chronic condition, research has shown that its impact on everyday life can be minimized through self-management. People who self-manage their hearing loss also experience greater satisfaction with hearing care and hearing technologies.

In the patients are joint decision makers, creating treatment plans that reflect their unique needs and desires. Patient collaboration in goal setting promotes greater self-efficacy and self-regulation. Self-efficacy involves the self-confidence to execute a behavior change. People with strong self-efficacy beliefs are more likely to persevere through challenges and to learn and regularly use new behaviors to manage their health condition. A vast body of literature indicates that people who have high self-efficacy for implementing new goals also have more successful outcomes.

References

Hickson, L., 2012. Defining a paradigm shift. *Seminars in Hearing*, 33(1), pp. 3–8, doi: 10.1055/ s-0032-1304722.

Ida Institute, 2010. I'd rather bring it out – up front – let people know it. Ida ethnographic films, Living Well series, New York, USA [online]. Available from: http://idainstitute.com/ toolbox/video_library/ethnographic_films/living_well_films/ [Accessed 16 March 2016].

MacDonald, G. and Jensen-Campbell, L. (Eds.), 2011. *Social pain, neuropsychological and health implications of loss and exclusion.* Washington, DC: American Psychological Association.

Manchaiah, V., Stephens, D., and Meredith, R., 2011. The patient journey of adults with hearing impairment: The patients' view. *Clinical Otolaryngology*, 36, pp. 227–234.

Manchaiah, V., 2013. Evaluating the process of change: Studies on patient journey, hearing disability acceptance and stages-of-change. Unpublished doctoral thesis. The Swedish Institute for Disability Research (SIDR), Linköping University, Sweden.

Prochaska, J. and Di Clemente, C., 1984. *The transtheoretical approach: Crossing traditional boundaries of therapy.* Homewood, IL: Dow/Jones Irwin.

Silvester, J., Patterson, F., Koczwara, A., and Ferguson, E., 2007. "Trust me …": Psychological and behavioral predictors of perceived physician empathy. *Journal of Applied Psychology*, 92(2), pp. 519–527.

Switankowsky, I., 2004. Empathy as a foundation for the biopsychosocial model of medicine. *Human Health Care*, 4(2), pp. E5–12.

Waller, D. and Sibbett, C. H. (Eds.), 2008. *Art therapy and cancer care.* Seoul, South Korea: HakJiSa Publisher/Oxford University Press.

Willett, J. and Deegan, M., 2001. Liminality and disability: Rites of passage and community in hypermodern society. *Disability Studies Quarterly*, 21(3), pp. 137–152.

Appendices

APPENDIX 1: BRIEF ICF CORE SETS FOR HEARING LOSS

ICF category (numeric code)	ICF category
Body functions	
b126	Temperament and personality functions
b140	Attention functions
b144	Memory functions
b152	Emotional functions
b210	Seeing functions
b230	Hearing functions
b240	Sensations associated with hearing and vestibular function
Body structures	
s110	Structure of brain
s240	Structure of external ear
s250	Structure of middle ear
s260	Structure of inner ear
Activities and participation	
d115	Listening
d240	Handling stress and other psychological demands
d310	Communicating – with – receiving spoken messages
d350	Conversation
d360	Using communication devices and techniques
d760	Family relationships
d820	School education
d850	Remunerative employment
d910	Community life

ICF category (numeric code)	ICF category
Environmental factors	
e125	Products and technology for communication
e250	Sound
e310	Immediate family
e355	Health professionals
e410	Individual attitudes of immediate family members
e460	Societal attitudes
e580	Health services, systems, and policies

APPENDIX 2: COMPREHENSIVE ICF CORE SETS FOR HEARING LOSS

ICF category (numeric code)	ICF category
Body functions	
b117	Intellectual functions
b126	Temperament and personality functions
b1300	Energy level
b1301	Motivation
b140	Attention functions
b144	Memory functions
b152	Emotional functions
b1560	Auditory perception
b1561	Visual perception
b164	Higher-level cognitive functions
b167	Mental functions of language
b210	Seeing functions
b2300	Sound detection
b2301	Sound discrimination
b2302	Localizations of sound source
b2304	Speech discrimination
b235	Vestibular functions
b240	Sensations associated with hearing and vestibular function
b280	Sensation of pain
b310	Voice functions
b320	Articulation functions
b330	Fluency and rhythm of speech functions
Body structures	
s110	Structure of brain
s240	Structure of external ear

ICF category (numeric code)	ICF category
s250	Structure of middle ear
s260	Structure of inner ear
s710	Structure of head and neck region

Activities and participation

d110	Watching
d115	Listening
d140	Learning to read
d155	Acquiring skills
d160	Focusing attention
d175	Solving problems
d220	Undertaking multiple tasks
d240	Handling stress and other psychological demands
d310	Communicating- with- receiving spoken messages
d315	Communicating- with- receiving- nonverbal messages
d330	Speaking
d3503	Conversing with one person
d3504	Conversing with many people
d355	Discussion
d360	Using communication devices and techniques
d440	Fine hand use
d470	Using transportation
d475	Driving
d620	Acquisition of goods and services
d660	Assisting others
d710	Basic interpersonal interactions
d720	Complex interpersonal interactions
d730	Relating with strangers
d740	Formal relationships
d750	Informal social relationships
d760	Family relationships
d770	Intimate relationships
d810	Informal training
d820	School education
d825	Vocational training
d830	Higher education
d840	Apprenticeship (work preparation)
d845	Acquiring, keeping, and terminating a job
d850	Remunerative employment
d855	Non-remunerative employment
d860	Basic economic transactions
d870	Economic self-sufficiency
d910	Community life
d920	Recreation and leisure
d930	Religion and spirituality
d940	Human rights
d950	Political life and citizenship

(continued)

ICF category (numeric code)	ICF category

Environmental factors

e115	Products and technology for personal use in daily living
e120	Products and technology for personal indoor and outdoor mobility and transportation
e125	Products and technology for communication
e130	Products and technology for education
e135	Products and technology for employment
e140	Products and technology for culture, recreation, and sport
e145	Products and technology for the practice of religion and spirituality
e150	Design, construction, and building products and technology of buildings for public use
e155	Design, construction, and building products and technology of buildings for private use
e225	Climate
e240	Light
e2500	Sound intensity
e2501	Sound quality
e310	Immediate family
e315	Extended family
e320	Friends
e325	Acquaintances, peers, colleagues, neighbors, and community members
e330	People in positions of authority
e335	People in subordinate positions
e340	Personal care providers and personal assistants
e345	Strangers
e350	Domesticated animals
e355	Health professionals
e360	Other professionals
e410	Individual attitudes of immediate family members
e415	Individual attitudes of extended family members
e420	Individual attitudes of friends
e425	Individual attitudes of acquaintances, peers, colleagues, neighbors, and community members
e430	Individual attitudes of people in positions of authority
e440	Individual attitudes of personal care providers and personal assistants
e445	Individual attitudes of strangers
e450	Individual attitudes of health professionals
e455	Individual attitudes of other professionals
e460	Societal attitudes
e465	Social norms, practices, and ideologies
e515	Architecture and construction services, systems, and policies
e525	Housing services, systems, and policies
e535	Communication services, systems, and policies
e540	Transportation services, systems, and policies

ICF category (numeric code)	ICF category
e545	Civil protection services, systems, and policies
e550	Legal services, systems, and policies
e555	Associations and organizational services, systems, and policies
e560	Media services, systems, and policies
e570	Social security services, systems, and policies
e575	General social support services, systems, and policies
e580	Health services, systems, and policies
e585	Education and training services, systems, and policies
e590	Labor and employment services, systems, and policies

INDEX

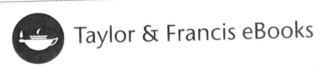

Taylor & Francis eBooks

Helping you to choose the right eBooks for your Library

Add Routledge titles to your library's digital collection today. Taylor and Francis ebooks contains over 50,000 titles in the Humanities, Social Sciences, Behavioural Sciences, Built Environment and Law.

Choose from a range of subject packages or create your own!

Benefits for you

>> Free MARC records
>> COUNTER-compliant usage statistics
>> Flexible purchase and pricing options
>> All titles DRM-free.

Benefits for your user

>> Off-site, anytime access via Athens or referring URL
>> Print or copy pages or chapters
>> Full content search
>> Bookmark, highlight and annotate text
>> Access to thousands of pages of quality research at the click of a button.

REQUEST YOUR **FREE** INSTITUTIONAL TRIAL TODAY

Free Trials Available
We offer free trials to qualifying academic, corporate and government customers.

eCollections – Choose from over 30 subject eCollections, including:

Archaeology	Language Learning
Architecture	Law
Asian Studies	Literature
Business & Management	Media & Communication
Classical Studies	Middle East Studies
Construction	Music
Creative & Media Arts	Philosophy
Criminology & Criminal Justice	Planning
Economics	Politics
Education	Psychology & Mental Health
Energy	Religion
Engineering	Security
English Language & Linguistics	Social Work
Environment & Sustainability	Sociology
Geography	Sport
Health Studies	Theatre & Performance
History	Tourism, Hospitality & Events

For more information, pricing enquiries or to order a free trial, please contact your local sales team:
www.tandfebooks.com/page/sales